Understanding and Managing Somatoform Disorders

A Guide For Clinicians

Understanding and Managing Somatoform Disorders

A Guide For Clinicians

FIRST EDITION

Anton Scamvougeras MBChB FRCPC
Andrew Howard MD FRCPC

AJ medical KS

Vancouver BC
Canada

Acknowledgements:
We would like to thank our colleagues in the UBC Neuropsychiatry team, for many years of rich dialogue, and without whom this book would not exist: Trevor Hurwitz, Leon Berzen, Marius Dimov, Magda Ilcewicz, Islam Hassan, Brenda Kosaka, Will Panenka, Robert Stowe, Joseph Tham, Peter Dawson, Annie Kuan, Gillian Brangham, Jackie Sabourin, Joyce Lacsamana, Cecilia Hynes, & Grace Wang. Thanks to medical students Nazia Hossain and Bennett Cheung who contributed to the appendices on pathophysiology and management. Thanks to Belinda Chen for her help in the early stages of the project, and to Annie Kuan, Caitlin Earle, & Jackie Sabourin for their help with final drafts. Thanks to Roger Frie for the title improvement, and to David Castle for the thoughtful encouragement. We are grateful to the patient who gave us permission to publish the illustration on pages 52-53.
We would like to thank our families - Margot, Adam, Jacob & Kate, and Jen, Lily & Ryan, for their love, support and good humour through this project.

Dedication:
This book is dedicated to our patients.

Disclosures:
The authors have no conflicts to declare.

Disclaimers:
The authors have worked to ensure that all information in this book is accurate at the time of publication and within general psychiatric and medical standards. Specific situations will likely arise that may require specific therapeutic responses that are not in this book. We strongly recommend that individuals seek and follow the advice of physicians directly involved in their care or in the care of a member of their family. Onus is on individual clinicians to ensure that standards of care are met within their jurisdiction of practice.

Contact:
Anton Scamvougeras: anton.scamvougeras@ubc.ca
Andrew Howard: andrew.howard@ubc.ca

Manufactured in Canada on FSC certified acid-free paper
First Edition

AJKS Medical is an imprint of AJKS Publishing, Vancouver BC Canada.

ISBN: 978-0-9952056-1-1

It is better to do something simple that is real.

- Bill Evans, jazz pianist

CONTENTS

The Authors:

Anton Scamvougeras MBChB FRCPC is a Consultant Neuropsychiatrist in the University of British Columbia Neuropsychiatry Program, and a Clinical Associate Professor in the UBC Department of Psychiatry, Vancouver, BC. He obtained his medical degree in Cape Town, South Africa, and then worked as a family physician in rural Canada before specializing in Psychiatry at McMaster University, Hamilton, Ontario, with fellowship studies in neurosciences, MRI, and research methodology. He has been at UBC since 1994, and has a special interest in understanding and helping individuals with severe Somatoform Disorders. He also runs the UBC Adult Tourette's Syndrome Clinic, assisting individuals with Tourette's and related conditions.

Andrew Howard MD FRCPC is a Consultant Neuropsychiatrist in the University of British Columbia Neuropsychiatry Program, and a Clinical Associate Professor in the UBC Department of Psychiatry, Vancouver, BC. He developed expertise in psychosomatic medicine, completing a psychology degree at Harvard, his MD at Queen's University, Kingston, Ontario, and psychiatry residency & neuropsychiatry fellowship at the University of British Columbia. He is the consultant psychiatrist to the Parkinson's and other movement disorders clinic, the Centre for Huntington's Disease, and to the deep brain stimulation program at UBC. He oversees the BC Neuropsychiatry Program's educational efforts serving medical students, residents, fellows and colleagues locally, nationally and internationally.

2 • SOMATOFORM DISORDERS

PREFACE

Who we are, and how we come to be helping individuals with Somatoform Disorders

The authors are members of a group of clinicians who treat individuals suffering from neuropsychiatric conditions. Most members of the group have a background in general psychiatry with subspecialization in neuropsychiatry. We work together as a team practising both inpatient and outpatient neuropsychiatry at UBC Hospital, University of British Columbia, Vancouver, Canada. A significant part of our work, up to 40% of our clinical time, is spent treating individuals suffering from severe Somatoform Disorders. Group members have between 5 and 30 years of experience working with this population. We began helping individuals with Somatoform Disorders largely by historic accident. Our founding member, Trevor Hurwitz, is both a neurologist and psychiatrist, and in the 1980's he began treating patients with Conversion Disorders who had been referred to him by his neurologist colleagues. Based on the work of earlier clinicians, he developed an approach to understanding and managing these conditions that is straightforward, sensible and effective, and which is largely based on his long-term follow-up of a cohort of severely affected patients (Hurwitz 2001, 2004). Each of us has learned to work with this model in subsequent years, in most cases adapting it to suit our individual clinical strengths, styles, and work methods. The work has resulted in a rich dialogue within our group, and our approach has been adapted and shaped by our discussions.

Using the general approach laid out in this text we have, as a group, now treated hundreds of patients with moderately severe to severe Somatoform Disorders, the majority with very good results. We believe that most mental health clinicians can adopt the strategies we employ to good effect. The approach has also proven to be useful to general practitioners and internists, who come into contact with a surprisingly high percentage of individuals with Somatoform Disorders in their practices.

What we have attempted in this text

We will describe a comprehensive, accessible approach to the understanding, assessment, and management of Somatoform Disorders. We share very specific aspects of our management techniques in a way that we believe will be beneficial to clinicians. Our aim is to help the reader find an approach that they can use to assist this population in their own clinical work. Parts of the text, particularly those regarding assessment, formulation, and management, are designed to give the reader something akin to the experience of being a member of our treating team, working with us to understand and help an individual with a Somatoform Disorder. The main body of the text serves as an introduction to our model and its practical application. That part of the text stands alone as a clinical guide. The appendices are designed for those interested in further background and context. A comprehensive discussion regarding the challenges of classification, which includes our recommended approach as well as a critique of DSM-5, appears as the first appendix, rather than earlier in the text, so as not to deflect from the clinical-guide focus of the main chapters. For similar reasons, literature reviews on pathophysiology and management also appear as appendices. We emphasize customizing care for each patient. Similarly, we believe that each clinician should adapt this general model to incorporate his or her own clinical style and strengths. For instance, different psychotherapeutic approaches may be used to assist an individual who has psychological distress as the predominant etiology of their somatization. The clinician should choose the psychotherapeutic techniques that make the most sense to them in that situation. In a similar fashion, there may be inter-clinician differences in the pharmacological choices used to treat neurovegetative features and psychiatric syndromes. The model tolerates this diversity in practice in some of the specifics of treatment, and that could be argued to be one of its strengths. The text is designed for clinicians who work with individuals with Somatoform Disorder or those who are in a position to begin such work but do not yet feel they have the tools or experience to do so. Our hope is that we will demystify this syndrome and make the challenge of assisting these individuals less daunting. We have been bold enough to call the book a 'First Edition', implying, somewhat playfully, that we believe that the text will prove to be sufficiently useful to merit further iterations. In this spirit we welcome suggestions, dialogue, and any useful criticism from fellow clinicians, researchers, and any other readers. Work with patients with Somatoform Disorders can be very taxing for the clinician. At the same time, successfully assisting individuals suffering from apparently treatment-resistant and puzzling conditions can be professionally gratifying. We hope that we will encourage more clinicians to join us in this work, and to engage in assisting the large population of individuals afflicted by these conditions, all of whom deserve good treatment. Our own clinical work has always been shaped primarily by the needs of our patients. Our model has itself been shaped over the years by the ways in which our patients have responded to our attempts to help them. In this regard, we have learnt much from them, we are grateful to them for that, and consequently, we dedicate this text to them.

Anton Scamvougeras
Andrew Howard

Vancouver, September 2018

References:

Hurwitz TA, Kosaka B: Primary psychiatric disorders in patients with conversion reactions. Journal of Depression & Anxiety 2001; 4:4-10

Hurwitz TA: Somatization and conversion disorder. Can J Psychiatry 2004; 49:172-8

CHAPTER 1

INTRODUCTION

Modern Medicine's 'Elephant In The Room'

Somatoform Disorders, conditions that occur when individuals express emotional distress indirectly as physical symptoms even when no physical pathology exists, are the 'elephant in the room' for modern medicine. We all know they are there, but by and large, we almost seem to pretend they are not. There is a remarkably high prevalence of these disorders in people seeking medical care, yet the conditions are strikingly under-identified and, more often than not, ignored. In primary care settings, Somatoform Disorders are the primary reason for presentation in 16 to 24 % of patients, depending on exact criteria used to identify the conditions (De Waal 2004). In the same settings, a significant but far lower percentage of individuals present overtly with psychiatric illnesses (5.5% depression, 4.0% anxiety disorder). This raises important questions about the form that emotional suffering takes in the community, and about the way in which people seek help for that distress.

Two important conclusions follow:

1. Significant emotional distress is being overlooked

Individuals will very often seek medical attention for emotional distress not via direct psychiatric complaints but rather indirectly, through somatoform symptoms. These patients are most often not identified as emotionally distressed, and their underlying suffering goes unidentified, unaddressed, and untreated.

2. Physical symptoms are being unnecessarily treated

A very significant proportion of individuals seeking primary medical care (about one in every five patients) have physical symptoms that are not caused by general medical conditions. Yet, the majority of those individuals will be diagnosed as suffering primarily physical ailments and receive treatments that are not directed at the cause of the symptoms. These treatments are often harmless, and in some cases may even indirectly and non-specifically help the individual. But in a significant percentage of cases, these treatments will be wasteful or even harmful. Misdirected therapies may be costly, may cause iatrogenic illness, and will distract proper attention away from the person's underlying distress.

An unfortunate collusion keeps somatoform conditions hidden

The reasons somatoform conditions go largely undetected are two-fold, the result of an unfortunate and unintended collaboration:

Firstly, the process whereby physical symptoms are generated by emotional distress is unconscious. The patient believes a physical illness is causing the problem, has little or no insight into the nature of the condition, and therefore understandably seeks, and even insists upon help for what is perceived to be a physical rather than psychiatric condition. In addition to this psychological process, the persistent and common stigma towards those presenting with overt manifestations of emotional or psychological distress compounds the difficulty in consciously identifying physical problems as psychiatric in origin.

Secondly, clinicians largely find these illnesses difficult to understand, and even more difficult to manage. Many physicians, even those specialized in psychiatry, will complete their training with the strong impression that Somatoform Disorder sufferers are a very challenging population to treat. Classification systems in use add to this general discomfort. They engender confusion in many clinicians, and have not translated into clinical benefits for patients. Furthermore, young doctors are unlikely in their training to have been exposed to the successful treatment of these conditions. This is partly because there are relatively few clinicians working specifically with these illnesses, and also because most often, successful treatment takes place over fairly lengthy longitudinal care, whereas trainees most often only observe brief cross-sectional periods in a patient's course. The understandable end result is that many physicians develop a career-long pessimism regarding these conditions. Thus, the patient's lack of insight and the clinician's discomfort and nihilism, collude to ensure that these conditions are more often than not overlooked.

Common, important, and treatable

Somatoform Disorders are common and important. By virtue of the very significant burden of suffering borne by patients and the consequences for their families and communities, these conditions are worthy of far more attention than they currently receive. When one considers the relative impact on communities in comparison to many other important diseases, one can easily make an argument for the need for specialized multidisciplinary clinics to assist citizens with somatoform conditions. Somatoform Disorders are treatable. We aim in the chapters ahead to lay out for clinicians a straightforward approach to understanding, assessing, and managing these conditions. We hope to show that using this framework makes them 'approachable', and that straightforward management built on that understanding more often than not assists those suffering from these conditions.

Recommended use of the term 'Somatoform Disorder' and our suggested system of classification

Even though not rigorously scientifically proven, we think that there is adequate evidence to believe that there exists a common process whereby emotional distress is expressed in the form of physical symptoms and signs. That process is referred to as 'somatization'.

We recommend naming a condition a 'Somatoform Disorder' in any clinical situation where physical symptoms and signs are judged, after thorough assessment, to be the result of underlying emotional distress rather than primary physical disease.

Further, as we do not see any evidence of any discernible etiological reason to separate somatoform presentations on the basis of whether the symptoms appear neurological or not, we collapse all somatoform syndromes (including conversion-type syndromes) into a single 'Somatoform Disorder' entity. Clinicians may still choose to refer to a somatoform syndrome with neurological signs as a 'Conversion Disorder', but we would still see that syndrome as a Somatoform Disorder (and would then describe the physical features in detail).

Thus, throughout the text, when we refer to a 'Somatoform Disorder', we are referring to conditions where any physical symptom or sign (neurological or non-neurological) is judged by the clinician, after adequate assessment, to be the result of underlying emotional distress rather than primary physical disease. As we are specific in the use of this name, we capitalize the first letters of the term throughout the text.

In the book we also suggest a straightforward descriptive system of classification that follows from our understanding of these conditions, that we believe is useful for clinicians and patients, and at the same time will be a sound foundation for research aimed at better understanding of these conditions. The approach is not unprecedented, and is partly based on earlier work of others. For an account of our suggested classification system and its use, see pp. 155-7, and also p. 63 & pp. 25-31.

We are aware that our position is at odds with some of the current trends in the understanding and classification of these conditions. But we believe the position will prove to be valid, and that many working in the field will see the benefits of this approach. For a thorough discussion of the challenges of classification, and for a critique of the DSM-5 approach, please see Appendix I (pp. 141-59).

Reference:

De Waal MW, Arnold IA, Eekhof JA, van Hemert AM: Somatoform disorders in general practice: prevalence, functional impairment and comorbidity with anxiety and depressive disorders. British Journal of Psychiatry 2004; 184:470-6

The following chapter presents an understanding to be used when assessing and helping individuals with Somatoform Disorders. A related consideration of the challenges of classifying somatoform conditions, including discussion of the APA's DSM-5, is covered in Appendix I: 'The Classification of Somatoform Disorders' (pp. 141-59).

CHAPTER 2

UNDERSTANDING SOMATOFORM DISORDERS

Clinical vignette: *A 35-year-old health care professional, living in rural Canada, was going through a very stressful period in his life. He felt ill-suited to his demanding job and stressed by a difficult relationship break-up. One of his symptoms was insomnia, and one night at 3 a.m. he sat up in bed feeling very emotionally distressed and agitated. He was experiencing intensely uncomfortable complex feelings of anxiety and sadness. He describes then having a remarkable experience: "Suddenly a calm came over me, and I felt everything was going to be okay... and that's when my body went crazy..." He instantly felt far less emotional distress, but from that moment on, he began to suffer a bizarre, non-anatomical, migratory pain syndrome, with severe pain that alternated each day from one side of the body to another in mirror image patterns. The pain was thereafter subject to much medical investigation and treatment. Remarkably, despite being able to give the above account, the patient's insight into the relationship between the pain and his emotions remained very limited.*

Human emotions are closely associated with distinct physical manifestations

Most obviously, consider the different facial expressions that we take on when we experience emotions such as fear, sadness or anger. In addition, each of those emotions is accompanied by other well known physical changes: anxiety with increased heart rate, tremulousness and pallor; sadness with slowness and slumped, contracted posture; anger with increased muscle tension, flushed facies and enlarged posture. These physical features can be argued to be as integral a part of the emotions as the mental experience of the emotions themselves. Thus, the idea of emotions having physical manifestations is not one that is foreign to us.

Emotional distress can be expressed as physical symptoms

This can happen through very direct physiological mechanisms, as in an individual who experiences tremulousness, quickened heart beat, and strange sensations over their chest and shoulders during a brief episode of intense anxiety. These symptoms are all direct effects of sympathetic nervous system activity. At other times the mechanism is less direct, as in a person who experiences weakness in an arm or an alteration of gait after a significant loss, or during an episode of untriggered endogenous depressed mood. More indirect still, individuals may experience symptoms such as constricted visual fields or a sense of deafness or an elaborate pain syndrome, in response to an altercation with a housemate, a threat of job loss, or the beginnings of neurochemical disturbance in, for instance, the hypomania of Bipolar Affective Disorder, the intense episodes of anxiety in Panic Disorder, or the depressed mood of an episode of Major Depression. At times a source of emotional distress may be obvious, at others, less clear.

Individuals respond in different ways to emotions, and to the physical manifestations of emotion

One person may be quick to interpret a fast heart-rate and tightened chest as symptoms of intense anxiety; another may experience and interpret the exact same symptoms as signs of cardiac disease and thus visit an emergency room. The latter individual may even go on to seek emergency care repeatedly, despite thorough assessments and reassurance from medical professionals that they suffer no sinister heart disease.

We don't yet fully understand the interpersonal differences in response, nor the exact mechanisms by which elaborate physical symptoms and signs emerge from underlying emotional distress. But we do know enough about this phenomenon to construct a useful framework to guide our clinical work and ongoing research enquiry, until we understand more.

Somatoform Disorders are characterized by symptoms and signs that appear to be physical in origin but which cannot be explained in terms of physical disease

Somatoform symptoms and signs, after thorough history, examination and necessary investigations, are found to be unrelated to demonstrable physical disease, or are far out of proportion to any identified disease.

Somatoform symptoms and signs are judged to be the result of the unconscious and involuntary physical expression of underlying emotional distress

These symptoms likely emerge when emotional distress is involuntarily and unconsciously expressed in the form of physical symptoms. This process is called 'somatization'. Evidence for the validity of the somatization process includes the non-physiological patterns of symptoms (they do not follow the patterns seen in well described diseases), the patterns of symptoms based on patient beliefs, the high rates of association of somatoform symptoms with overt emotional distress, the many persuasive clinical examples of 'conversion' of mental distress into physical symptoms & signs, the longitudinal natural history of these conditions (with only very small percentages revealing causative underlying sinister tissue pathology over time), and the positive responses to therapies when a somatoform model is assumed.

The exact mechanism whereby somatoform symptoms appear has not yet been conclusively and scientifically demonstrated. (For a review of current evidence of neurobiological correlates, see Appendix III, pp. 165-175.)

Somatization is initially adaptive in that the immediate resultant physical distress is less threatening and more tolerable than the immediate experience of the direct emotional distress

This process is well illustrated by the clinical vignette that started this chapter. Somatization can be seen as an 'ego defence' in that the process protects the individual's 'self' from the immediate and direct experience of emotional distress. The experience of emotional dysphoria is eased by the emergence of physical symptoms. This is known as 'primary gain' - the 'gain' being the decrease in emotional distress.

The individual described in the vignette shares with us the moment and the experience of primary gain. He describes the very instant of the 'conversion' of symptoms from the emotional to the physical. For him, the relief from the intense emotional distress would appear, on some level, to be 'worth' the considerable physical suffering. This may seem unusual to the objective observer, but that observer is likely to be underestimating the intensity of the dysphoria that the patient faces. The patient gains relief from this intense psychological discomfort by way of the somatization defence. For the individual who is experiencing this psychic pain, the complex unconscious emotional-physical bargaining results in a deal that would seem, at least at first, to be a good one.

The majority of individuals with Somatoform Disorders do not have as distinct an onset of their symptoms as the man above recounts. The onset may be anything from very rapid to insidious. But we believe the process is essentially the same.

All somatoform conditions have two components: the underlying emotional distress, and the psychogenic physical symptoms and signs that are an unconscious expression of that distress

It is extremely important to keep this in mind. To lump together groups of individuals with similar psychogenic physical manifestations is to forget that they may each have very different underlying forms of dysphoria. And when attempting to help people suffering from these conditions, it is extremely important to customize your understanding and approach to each individual's combination of underlying emotional distress and physical manifestations.

The physical symptoms and signs in Somatoform Disorders can take many forms

Common somatoform symptoms are traditionally divided into pseudo-neurological symptoms and those from other systems of the body. Conversion Disorder classically includes somatoform symptoms that appear neurological such as: paralysis; loss of vision or sensation; convulsions; spells of altered consciousness; involuntary movements; or problems with walking, speech, or swallowing (including globus hystericus, a sense of a mass in the throat). Other somatoform symptoms involve non-neurological systems and include: pain all over the body or in specific regions such as the head, arms, legs, joints, muscles, chest, back, pelvis, genitals, face or jaw; chronic fatigue; intermittent abdominal discomfort or other gastrointestinal tract dysfunction such as nausea with or without vomiting and food intolerance; urinary difficulties and symptoms of frequent urinary infections; sexual dysfunction; pain with intercourse; dizziness; breathlessness or rapid breathing; and a sense of a strong, faster, or irregular heartbeat.

The separation of Conversion Disorder symptoms from other psychogenic symptoms that is emphasized in some classification systems is most likely not going to turn out to be based on valid differences in pathogenicity. Many patients have symptoms on both sides of this divide. All of these symptoms are believed to be expressions of underlying emotional distress.

Somatoform Disorders vary in severity of physical symptoms and in chronicity of course

The symptoms vary from very mild to very severe, and may be fleeting and transitory, or become chronic and entrenched, with some even lasting many decades.

There are large numbers of individuals in the general population experiencing somatoform symptoms at any one time

About 16-24% of individuals seeking help from primary medical clinics do so because of a somatoform condition (Fink 1999, De Waal 2004). That number may be as high as 35% in neurology clinics (Snijders 2004, Stone 2009).

The majority of minor somatoform symptoms are never identified nor labeled as somatoform

They either resolve unattended or resolve coincidentally after first step treatment for a presumed physical condition. In these cases we would imagine that the underlying emotional distress is, like the physical symptoms, fleeting and relatively mild. These forms of mild transitory symptoms are perhaps more likely to be the result of psychologically generated emotional distress, as one sees in response to temporary environmental stressors. Some biologically driven causes of transitory emotional distress, as one may see in Panic Disorder, may also initially present with mild and transitory somatoform reactions. We expect them to have a high chance of recurring in those cases, as the underlying causes of emotional distress tend to persist and recur.

Clinical Vignette: *The CEO of a large North American corporation described her own somatoform experience in a New York Times biographical sketch: "About 5 years ago I was the human resources manager for a large well known firm in North America, commuting from one large city to another. I reached a point in my life when I did not feel well physically. I was pushing myself too much. I ended up going to the hospital one night because I felt so horrible. I had numbness in my arm. That really scared me. The doctor said it was built up stress." The CEO went on to describe changing her lifestyle, feeling less "stressed", and the physical symptoms resolved (Spiers-Lopez, 2004).*

These kinds of short-lived somatoform symptoms likely occur very commonly in the community, most often without even being formally considered somatoform conditions.

At the more severe end of the spectrum, individuals are disabled completely and for many years by conditions that may include symptoms of pain, frequent nonepileptic seizures, movement disorders, blindness, deafness, mutism, dysphasias and even quadriplegia.

Clinical Vignette: *A 65-year-old woman presented with a 7-year history of unexplained abdominal symptoms. Further discussion revealed that, starting in her twenties, she had suffered a series of unexplained medical syndromes, each of which incapacitated her for many years. These included a syndrome of severe leg-weakness and fatigue, a long period of suffering from unusual visual disturbances, a period of suffering seizure-like spells, and a lengthy period with imbalance and gait disturbance. Thorough investigation of each of these syndromes had not revealed any identifiable medical cause. She had not experienced any significant amount of time symptom-free for over 40 years. After thorough assessment and the conclusion that she was suffering a chronic protean Somatoform Disorder, she responded well to education, psychotherapy and pharmacotherapy, and her quality of life improved.*

Somatoform symptoms are based on the individual's understanding of body physiology and disease mechanisms

A Somatoform Disorder reflects the sufferer's understanding of their own physiology and how a disease should affect their body. As a result, symptoms and signs do not typically fit the classic patterns of presentations seen with typical illness pathophysiology.

For example, basic understanding of contralateral neurological relationships are now common in the general population, based on education and experience of relatives with strokes and so forth. Thus it is not uncommon to see patients with unilateral psychogenic facial or cranial symptoms with corresponding contralateral peripheral symptoms:

> **Clinical Vignette:** *A 58-year-old man slipped at work, fell backwards and sustained a mild blow to the back of his head. He was briefly stunned but did not lose consciousness. Neurological examination and MRI brain scan were normal. Over the following three months he developed a more and more complicated set of physical symptoms that included left sided headache, twitching movements in the muscles around his left eye, an intermittent tremor in his right hand, and adduction myoclonic jerks of his legs. Further investigation including ambulatory EEG revealed no evidence of partial seizures or any gross demonstrable pathology. His movements all decreased or stopped with distraction, and increased greatly when his attention was drawn to them. He explained that the left-sided periorbital movements and the right hand tremor were related because "the left side of the brain controls the right side of the body".*

In a related fashion, the splitting of vibration sense over the same bone at the midline in individuals with psychogenic unilateral sensory deficits is an example of a common misunderstanding of body physiology leading to a similar psychogenic sign occurring across individuals. If a neurologist were to develop a Somatoform Disorder, one would expect a particularly complex presentation.

Once somatoform symptoms are initiated, secondary physical phenomena can reinforce the condition

Somatoform pain or weakness can lead to atypical use of part of the body, that itself can then lead to musculoskeletal symptoms: pain from joint or soft tissue inflammation, muscle spasm from defensive bracing, and discomfort from abnormal gait or posture. Thus, there may be peripheral evidence of this atypical use, such as edema in a psychogenically paralyzed limb. Dysfunction and disability, however, always remain disproportionally larger than any demonstrable peripheral tissue pathology.

Habit can perpetuate the symptoms

Somatoform symptoms and signs are established as a result of underlying emotional distress. They are most often perpetuated by ongoing emotional distress, but if the underlying emotional distress settles, some symptoms, signs and related behaviours may continue, despite the absence of an ongoing primary emotional 'need' for the symptoms. Physical habit, as with a gait disturbance, or psychological habit, as with episodic symptoms triggered by specific circumstance, may play a part.

Social habit and expectations may also work against an individual, and delay resolution of physical symptoms and signs. It may seem socially unacceptable for an individual who has, say, required a wheelchair for two years, and the support of others, to then be seen independently walking around the house or the neighbourhood.

Somatoform symptoms and signs are produced by unconscious and involuntary mechanisms

The symptoms emerge without conscious intent on the part of the individual. The person's experience of the symptoms is predominantly physical. They feel the pain, experience the deficits, and are physically affected by the symptoms as if they were the result of physical disease. They most often have little or no insight into the mechanism of the condition.

A minority of patients display classic 'la belle indifference', where they show apparent lack of concern about the symptoms; they experience the physical symptoms in a detached fashion, sometimes almost as though they don't actually own the body which the symptoms are afflicting. This is sometimes misinterpreted by others to represent a lack of motivation to recover. 'La belle indifference' is relatively uncommon. What is more common is for individuals to express concern about their symptoms and to seek medical care out of that concern.

The patient, as a result of the unconscious & involuntary nature of the condition, believes he or she is ill in this fashion

The patient suffering a somatoform symptom experiences it as entirely real; their core experience is of the physical symptom and the resultant disability. In fact, patients can hold tightly to their beliefs that they are physically unwell even in the face of unquestionable evidence to the contrary (test results, expert opinions, reversibility demonstrated by narcoanalysis or psychiatric treatment).

This belief distinguishes the disorder from conditions where symptoms are consciously fabricated, namely factitious disorders and malingering. In factious disorders, an individual consciously induces physical symptoms for reasons of obtaining medical attention or other attention of some sort. There is no obvious material gain. In malingering, an individual consciously induces physical symptoms for reasons of obtaining material gain which may include substances, financial gain, avoidance of studies, work or military duty. They are at all times aware of the goal and of the nature of the deceit.

Some patients may note that symptoms could be 'stress' related

A minority of those affected with Somatoform Disorders may volunteer a relationship between emotional distress (commonly described by them as 'stress') and their physical symptoms. They may even hypothesize that 'stress' may have caused some of the symptoms. This subgroup of individuals is further along in their steps to gain insight into their condition, and those sorts of interpersonal differences are noted in assessment and lead to variations in formulation and management.

Somatoform symptoms usually worsen when attention is focused on them but improve with distraction, thus they may be mistakenly thought to be voluntarily induced

As the symptoms are the result of the individual's cognitively held beliefs, they are most prominent when attention is drawn to them. Conversely, the symptoms and signs are less prominent (but, out of habituation, almost always still present to some degree) when the individual's attention is spontaneously or intentionally distracted. Thus, signs may be seen to improve when an individual is forced to perform a task that is incompatible with the maintenance of the symptom. For instance, beating out an irregular pattern with one hand may alter a psychogenic tremor in another limb.

The pattern of worsening of signs with attention and improvement of signs with distraction is an indication that the syndrome is psychogenic, *not* an indication that the affected individual is consciously producing the symptoms.

Decreased conscious awareness decreases symptoms

Decreased consciousness or decreased attentiveness brought on by sleep, somnolence, sedation, inebriation, delirium, or post-electroconvulsive therapy confusion, may result in symptoms becoming less prominent. The disinhibition induced by a sodium amytal interview (or other medications such as parenteral benzodiazepines used for narcoanalysis or sedation) is designed to elicit this phenomenon and can be used for diagnostic and/or treatment purposes (see pp. 102-5). Video of an individual suffering psychogenic symptoms, with their consent, while they are asleep, can perform a similar role, showing movement or range of motion in a psychogenically 'paralyzed' limb that is incapable of being voluntarily moved when the patient is fully conscious. Other forms of decreased levels of consciousness can also cause a temporary remission of symptoms:

> **Clinical Vignette:** *A 25-year-old man developed a psychogenic speech and gait disturbance over the six months following a minor head injury. During amytal interview the symptoms disappeared entirely but returned once the acute effects of the amytal wore off. He was judged to be suffering an underlying severe major depression. When all other psychological and pharmacological treatments failed to help his symptoms, he elected to attempt a course of electroconvulsive therapy. For up to one hour after each treatment, while in a state of post-ictal confusion, the symptoms resolved completely and he was able to talk and walk fluently. In each instance, as his awareness returned and his confusion cleared, the symptoms reconstituted. He*

did not respond to the ECT trial in any sustained fashion, and his condition remains treatment resistant years later.

Some individuals are more prone to somatize emotional distress

Why would one individual express emotional distress directly, but another individual express it indirectly as a physical symptom? We do not yet know the full answer to that question, the best we can do is to look at evidence from empirically associated factors, and theories regarding interpersonal differences regarding the tendency to somatize.

We know that certain individuals are at higher risk. Those from lower socioeconomic groups, with less education, who have experienced physical or sexual abuse, who have a neurological illness or a psychiatric illness, and a family history of somatization, are all more predisposed. Patients with depression and neurodegenerative conditions are at increased risk. The human tendency to somatize is universal, but some cultures may somatize more, and some patterns of somatization are specific to some cultures (Kirmayer 1998). People who have more difficulty recognizing and reporting their own feelings (individuals referred to as 'alexithymic') are predisposed to manifesting somatoform symptoms (Mattila 2008). If negative emotions do emerge in these individuals, they usually do so in an indirect fashion. The question: "How is your mood?" may be answered: "I'm tired." Families and individuals who favour reporting physical distress rather than emotional distress, even as a lexical habit (e.g. 'that makes me sick'), may be at increased risk. Somatoform disorder patients report higher incidences of paranoid, dependent, and obsessive-compulsive personality traits. Whether these traits are due to common childhood pathogenic experiences, or themselves put patients at risk, is unclear.

Clinical Vignette: *A 50-year-old man recalled that as a boy, he had felt neglected and rejected by his parents, but vividly recalled one incident where he was hospitalized and was well cared for by nursing staff. When he became ill as a young adult, his wife stepped into an ardent caregiving role. Multiple somatic complaints had led to more than ten years of serial surgeries and other treatments, all without benefit. He was admitted for assessment of apparent complex somatoform illness. On seeing his physician enter his hospital room one morning, he greeted him with: "Welcome to my one true abode!"*

An individual such as this patient, with dependent personality traits, may be predisposed to seek nurturing in a round-about way from medical caregivers and other people in their lives. We should keep in mind that psychological factors such as these could sustain or even cause a somatoform condition.

'Suggestion' is the process whereby interpersonal interaction, or another form of event, controls or shapes the thoughts, feelings or behaviours of an individual. There is evidence that patients with somatoform conditions are more suggestible than people in the general community. They have been shown to be more easily hypnotizable and more prone to dissociation (Simeon 2008). However, these differences tend to extinguish when one controls for variation in levels of anxiety and depression, so it is not clear that suggestibility is of utmost importance in determining whether a person develops a Somatoform Disorder or not. Patients with somatoform conditions do not appear to dissociate more than other psychiatric patients with similar severities of psychopathology. Suggestibility may shape the physical expression of the underlying psychological or emotional distress in somatoform patients rather than serving as a direct causation. Nonetheless, there are certain scenarios where it is striking how symptoms appear to result from something suggested, as in the following account:

Clinical Vignette: *A 29-year-old man working in an industrial plant grabbed a live cable with his right hand, resulting in a period of electrocution during which he yelled out and convulsed his upper body in a rhythmical fashion. His alarmed colleagues frantically struggled to switch off the power, taking 30 seconds to do so. Three female co-workers, who routinely worked next to him and were well known to the man, were particularly deeply emotionally traumatized by the experience of watching him suffer. They instantly became classically hysterical, moving their upper bodies and arms in high amplitude tremor, and yelling out, in the same way that their co-worker had done during electrocution. They continued to behave in this fashion throughout an ambulance ride to the local ER. They all settled rapidly in the ER, management being that of oral rapid acting benzodiazepine and, just as important, separating the three individuals such that they no longer acted as sources of suggestion to each other. The man fortunately suffered no immediate or delayed ill effects from the electrocution.*

Various mechanisms may determine the choice of specific somatoform symptom or sign

Symbolism

Earlier understandings of somatoform symptoms emphasized the psychological 'meaning' or 'symbolism' of the patient's symptom or clinical signs. An example would be an angry individual with violent intent developing a psychogenic paralysis of their arm, so as to make the feared violence less possible. On occasion one will see patients where such mechanisms may be at play, and that conclusion would shape the clinician's approach to management of the emotional distress and the physical symptom itself. Far more often, however, symbolism does not appear to be involved in the development of somatoform symptoms.

Physiological effects of emotion

Some symptoms may be a result of a physiological disturbance cued directly by the nature of the emotional distress. Anxiety can by direct neurological or less direct humoral effects, cause well-known physical symptoms that may include a mass-like sensation in the throat ('globus hystericus'), palpitations, tightness across the chest, tremor, increased muscle tension, fatigue, nausea, abdominal discomfort, and dizziness. Similarly, depressed mood can cause motor slowing and fatigue. These physical symptoms can themselves become the focus of presentation or act as a nidus for a more complex somatoform illness. Amplified and distorted symptoms may then become sustained, and dissociated from the purely physiological symptoms of emotion.

Misinterpretation of normal physiology

Some somatoform symptoms may be cued by 'normal' physical symptoms and body sensations that are then misinterpreted as pathological. This would include phenomena such as fleeting discomfort on pressure points, brief light-headedness on standing, mild shortness of breath on ascending stairs, or normal sensations of bowel physiology.

Elaboration upon injury

Some symptoms may be triggered by injury. Initial limited symptoms become more elaborate, more severe, more widespread as a result of somatoform mechanisms. A trivial blow to the head causes minor scalp discomfort but then becomes a psychogenic head tremor; or a minor focal peripheral injury amplifies to become a regional pain syndrome.

Cued by symptoms of another illness
The physical symptom of a peripheral disease process may act as a nidus around which a somatoform condition develops, for instance: an attack of multiple sclerosis affecting foot sensation that becomes a psychogenic limb paralysis.

Modelled on another illness
Somatoform symptoms may be modelled on another illness from which the person suffers. An example of this would be psychogenic non-epileptic seizure-like episodes in a person who also has epilepsy.

Modelled on illnesses in others
Some symptoms and signs may be modelled on illnesses observed in others, for instance an ill family member or a co-patient on a ward.

Cued by suggestion
Still others may seem cued by suggestion:

> **Clinical Vignette:** *A 32-year-old woman in a difficult romantic relationship, and suffering from chronic Hepatitis C, was experiencing emotional distress with depressed and anxious mood. One morning she was in her kitchen making a cup of tea, and feeling particularly dysphoric. As she shut a cupboard, a housemate - themselves disgruntled - angrily snapped: "Why are you always making so much noise? Are you deaf or something?" Thereafter, the woman started questioning her hearing ability and came to the conclusion that her hearing was indeed deteriorating. She then noted a rapid and steady decrease in hearing acuity and over the following week she developed complete psychogenic deafness as well as the high-pitched nasal speech characteristic of those deaf from birth. She was referred for assessment by her hepatologist. After thorough assessment, hearing and speech returned to normal after formulation and use of amytal interview.*

Chance
Some symptoms may be determined in an almost random fashion, by chance alone. Perhaps during a period of intense dysphoria an individual stumbles and then develops a gait disturbance, or drops something and develops hand weakness, or experiences a mild abdominal sensation and develops an abdominal pain syndrome.

Symptoms created via possible specific neurobiological effects
A few symptoms of somatoform presentation are seen across many individuals in a strikingly similar fashion, and suggest an underlying predisposition to showing emotional distress in stereotyped physical ways. There is a possibility that yet unknown specific neurobiological factors determine these symptom choices. For instance, psychogenic concentric contraction of the visual fields ('tunnel vision') is not uncommon (see p. 59). This symptom, which does not obviously appear to be cognitively or socially cued, raises interesting questions. Is it possible that some physiological manifestation of anxiety or some other dysphoria cues the individual to experience a concentric shrinking of their visual fields, even though the perpetuation of such a deficit is clearly non-neurological? Or is there some other yet unknown specific neurobiological or cognitive mechanism at work? Is psychogenic tunnel-vision a valid marker for a subgroup of somatoform patients that are pathophysiologically similar in other ways?

Use a straightforward approach to understand Somatoform Disorders by asking two central questions:

1. Is a somatoform process causing the illness?

We by default presume that most individuals experience and communicate significant emotional distress in a relatively direct fashion. People vary in their ability to do this, even within the typical range:

Emotional distress -> Emotional symptoms

A sizeable minority express emotional distress indirectly in the form of physical symptoms:

Emotional distress -> (somatization) -> Physical symptoms

If this process is occurring, the symptoms are somatoform. They may be entirely somatoform in nature, or the somatoform process may be amplifying more minor underlying symptoms of physical disease.

If the patient has symptoms and signs that after very thorough assessment are not adequately explained by any demonstrated underlying medical condition, and that are clearly and consistently atypical and more likely a product of a belief that the individual is ill rather than the fact that he or she is ill, then they are suffering a somatoform condition.

If the severity of the somatoform symptoms are significantly interfering with the individual's function, and/or are causing them to seek medical assistance, they have then crossed a threshold where we can say that they have a condition which merits description as a Somatoform Disorder.

2. If so, what is the nature and cause of the underlying emotional distress?

We are then led to ask:
What is the nature of that underlying emotional distress?
In other words, what is the nature of the 'engine' that is driving the illness? We are very aware that answering this question is often a complex challenge.

For the sake of guiding the patient's understanding and our own management, we heuristically break down the source of the conceptualized emotional distress into two types. The first is associated with psychiatric syndromes and thought to be the result of dysregulation of biochemistry in neurological circuitry. The second is caused by psychological conflicts that the individual is experiencing within his or her current life circumstances.

So, we suggest making a straightforward attempt at trying to subdivide the sources of distress as follows:

Psychiatric and Psychological underpinnings

(a) 'Psychiatric' causes of distress.

By this we mean relatively severe illness characterized by neurochemical brain disturbances and brain circuit dysregulation. These illnesses include many that would merit a DSM diagnosis: Panic Disorder, Major Depression, Bipolar Affective Disorder with or without active mania or hypomania, various other psychotic illnesses such as Schizophrenia or Delusional Disorders, as well as Substance Abuse and Post Traumatic Stress Disorder. These disorders can all express themselves in the form of predominantly somatoform presentations. In these illnesses, neurovegetative changes (such as disturbed sleep, poor energy, low appetite, absent libido) are common, even where the emotional distress is less obvious and largely somatized.

> **Clinical Vignette:** *A 63-year-old retired emergency services worker was referred with a 12-month history of intermittent speech disturbance, which had initially been feared to represent strokes. These episodes would occur a few times a week, and last a few minutes. Neurological examination and investigations had proven to be normal. History revealed that for ten years prior to the onset of the speech disturbance, the patient had experienced intermittent episodes of dizziness and nausea that would require him to lie on the ground and be administered IM dimenhydrinate. These episodes were replaced by the intermittent speech disturbance episodes, and had not reoccurred. Going further back in the history, it became apparent that the very first episode of dizziness had come on when he was vividly reminded of a very traumatic work experience, in which he had to deal with a dismembered body after a horrifying accident. On recounting this incident, he appeared terrified and distraught, as though experiencing it again. He was found to be suffering symptoms compatible with PTSD, the severe distress from which had been somatized into one physical syndrome and then another. He gained much relief from education regarding the nature of his condition, cognitive behavioural therapy, and concurrent pharmacotherapy (Wald 2004).*

(b) 'Psychological' causes of distress.

By this we mean there is an untenable interaction between the individual's psychological 'self' ('who they are'; their temperament, their character, their personality), and their current life circumstances. This includes causes of distress during which coping mechanisms are overwhelmed, and reserves are depleted. There is a great deal of interpersonal variation in how individuals respond to different stressors. Understanding the contribution of this component calls for a thorough, and often longitudinal, psychological assessment of the patient.

We are aware that conceptualizing this 'Psychiatric' and 'Psychological' approach to the understanding of the emotional 'engine' is perhaps going to seem outrageously simplistic and excessively dichotomous to some observers. Yes, there is overlap in those two categories. Yes, distress in one can beget distress in the other; their interrelationships are remarkably complex. And, yes, they are all the result of, on some level, biological brain processes. But we do believe that this is a valid distinction to make. In fact, it is the distinction that medical professionals attempt to make all around the world, tens of thousands of times per day, when they try to understand whether individuals presenting with overt emotional distress are doing so for endogenous biological reasons, or as a response that is appropriate, for that individual, to the challenges presented by their environment. Thus:

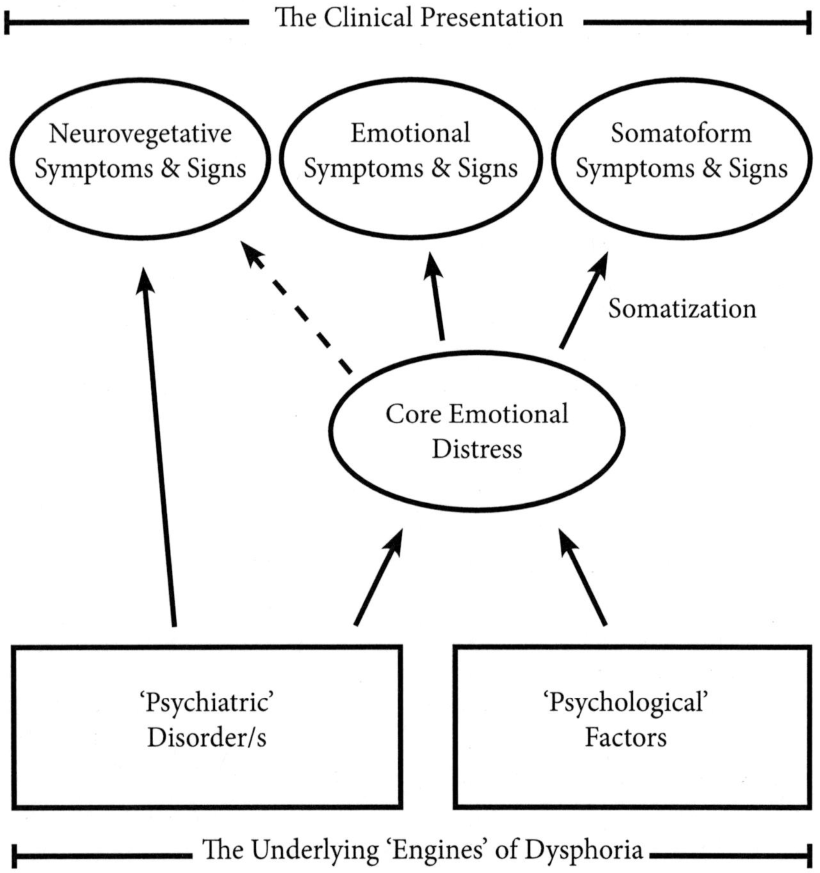

This very straightforward approach makes good clinical sense. We believe that it is a 'valid' model, in that it is broadly in keeping with the processes that are at play in the pathogenesis and pathophysiology of

Somatoform Disorders. It results in a logical way of understanding these conditions. It leads to an organized and flexible approach to management. It still allows for the all important customization of understanding for each individual sufferer. Each patient is different regarding the nature of their underlying emotional distress, and in the physical manifestations thereof. This approach to understanding allows for the development of unique interventions with each patient, depending on their specific needs.

Describing and Documenting The Diagnosis

For the purpose of clearly describing and documenting your diagnosis, use the following multidimensional, reductionistic method:

Call the condition a 'Somatoform Disorder', which is an accurate label:
'Somatoform Disorder'
(present if apparent physical symptoms and signs are judged, after thorough assessment, to be the result of underlying emotional distress rather than primary physical disease)

Then describe the physical somatoform symptoms and signs:
1. **Physically manifesting as:** ______________________
(list and describe all of the physical somatoform symptoms and signs)

Then describe your current understanding of the nature of the emotional distress, breaking that down as best as possible:

2. **Probable cause/s of underlying emotional distress:**

(a) **Psychiatric syndrome:** ______________________
As evidenced by: ______________________
(list psychiatric symptoms and signs, including those pertaining to mood, anxiety, thought form, thought content, attention, motivation, perception, behaviour; as well as neurovegetative features such as sleep disturbance, appetite change, weight change, low energy/fatigue, decreased libido, psychomotor agitation/slowing)

(b) **Psychological contributors:** ______________________
As evidenced by: ______________________
(psychological features including developmental factors, personality,

coping style, conflicts, current circumstances, current stressors)

Thus a diagnostic template would look like this:

'Somatoform Disorder'
1. Physically manifesting as: ______________________
2. Probable cause/s of underlying emotional distress:
(a) Psychiatric syndrome: ______________________
As evidenced by: ________________________
(b) Psychological contributors: ____________________
As evidenced by: ____________________________

See Appendix I : 'On the Classification of Somatoform Disorders' (pp.141-59) for further discussion and context for this recommended approach.

The suggested approach offers a framework around which a customized understanding and flexible plan of management can be developed

This approach allows for a broad valid understanding of the somatoform process, while still emphasizing the importance of customizing a specific understanding for each individual. The approach we suggest is, at its core, very straightforward, but it should not be misunderstood as being unduly simplistic. It supplies a skeleton around which a more complex customized understanding and flexible plan of management can be developed for each patient. Such a plan takes into account the specific physical, psychiatric and psychological factors affecting the illness in each patient. Until there is good biological evidence for subgroups or clinical evidence that a more complex categorization will allow for more effectively targeted management, we would argue that this straightforward model and approach makes the most sense.

The core disorder is the underlying emotional distress; the somatic manifestations are secondary

This is a crucial and central point in understanding these disorders. The emotional distress is the primary condition, and the somatoform symptoms and signs are a manifestation of that underlying cause. Together they make up the somatoform syndrome. The precise manifestation of the physical distress is almost always less important than the emotional source and the individual's beliefs about their illness.

The prognosis is more closely related to the prognosis of the cause of the underlying emotional distress, than to any characteristics of the physical symptoms

The treatability of the condition is closely related to the treatability of the underlying cause of the emotional distress. Although chronicity or the extent of physical symptoms may suggest a more intractable disorder, the overall prognosis is far less closely determined by the physical symptoms than by the nature of the dysphoria.

The following vignette demonstrates how the severity of physical presentation does not necessarily predict for poor prognosis:

> **Clinical Vignette:** *A 19-year-old woman became emotionally distressed when her siblings started leaving the home to socialize with peers in ways that she felt socially ill equipped to emulate. She started experiencing episodes of a sensation of facial heat and leg weakness. The leg weakness progressed to the point that her parents took her to a local ER. She was admitted, and over 6 months she progressed to a state of complete quadriplegia, requiring total care for a further 9 months. She was admitted for a thorough assessment for Somatoform Disorder, and returned to baseline function after 2 months of intense multidisciplinary management. She remains well twenty years later, having experienced no episodes of recurrence.*

In the above example, an individual with an extreme physical disability proves to have a very good prognosis. In contrast to this example, there are many instances in which a less severe symptom, for instance a weak arm, resulting from a more intractable cause of underlying dysphoria such as lifelong psychological distress, will respond far less well to similarly ardent therapy.

Cogniform symptoms are the cognitive equivalent of physical somatoform symptoms

Cogniform symptoms are cognitive deficits driven by a process similar to that which produces the physical symptoms in somatoform conditions

(Delis 2007). In this case, emotional distress is defended against by the emergence of psychogenic cognitive deficits. The patient complains of some form of cognitive symptom, most commonly memory deficits and problems with attention. This occurs in the face of underlying normal cognitive function. There is no typical pattern of a dementing illness.

Cogniform symptoms and signs should be differentiated from those seen in the pseudodementia of depression, where biochemical dysfunction leads to actual psychomotor slowing, which directly affects concentration, memory and other cognitive functions. Cogniform symptoms may occur without the neurovegetative changes of depression, or are out of proportion to that which one would expect from the degree of depression or anxiety. Cogniform symptoms are often seen as part of a constellation of psychogenic symptoms in a patient with a complex somatoform disorder and, less often, they are the primary presenting complaint.

Cogniform symptoms should be approached as somatoform symptom equivalents. They can be managed using similar principles to those described for physical symptoms. Perhaps at some point in the future these conditions will be collapsed, and we will be referring to overarching 'psychogenic syndromes', which cover both physical and cognitive manifestations of indirectly expressed emotional distress. Until then, include cogniform symptoms when considering the spectrum of symptoms that may result from a somatization type process.

More similar than different: Fibromyalgia, Chronic Fatigue Syndrome, Irritable Bowel Syndrome, Seronegative Lyme's Disease, Multiple Chemical Sensitivity, and various other medically unexplained syndromes

There exists a group of medical conditions, common in the general community, that are quite likely in most sufferers to be misunderstood Somatoform Disorders. These conditions include Fibromyalgia, Chronic Fatigue Syndrome, Irritable Bowel Syndrome, Seronegative Lyme's Disease, non-cardiac chest pain, temporomandibular joint dysfunction, various environmental sensitivity syndromes, and others. There are numerous less common syndromes such as presumed heavy metal poisoning that could also be understood to be members of this group. People carrying these diagnoses, which are almost always chronic, often experience a great burden of suffering and may be severely disabled for many years by the associated symptoms. In these conditions there is no consistent, demonstrated tissue pathology to explain signs or symptoms, yet it is commonly presumed that they are the result of peripheral, non-brain-based, as yet undescribed tissue pathology. Many individuals with persistent post-concussive syndromes after trivial or minor head injuries are likely suffering somatoform conditions.

Crucially, there is substantial overlap in these conditions. Symptoms such as fatigue, sleep disturbance, decreased concentration, decreased motivation, pain, anxiety, and variations in mood, are common across each of the syndromes. Indeed, there is evidence that these syndromes are a great deal more similar than they are different (Wessely 1999, Aaron 2001, Aggarwal 2006). A study of interrelationships among 9 conditions (chronic fatigue syndrome, low back pain, irritable bowel syndrome, chronic tension headache, fibromyalgia, temporomandibular joint disorder, major depression, panic attacks, and PTSD) in a large sample (3982 twins) showed comorbidity far exceeding chance expectations (Schur 2007).

The recommended and most effective treatments for many of these conditions have substantial overlap with those that are useful in somatoform conditions. For instance, moderate exercise and tricyclic antidepressants are commonly recommended for Fibromyalgia and Chronic Fatigue Syndrome, even though it is often postulated that the medications are working at a peripheral level.

There is a high likelihood that these diagnoses are unconsciously being used as a more palatable way of supporting and treating what are actually underlying somatoform conditions. The reluctance of patients and medical caregivers to more openly explore the possibility of emotional distress as the primary driver for these conditions reflects again the broad stigma that our society still harbours towards mental illness.

If these conditions are indeed valid discrete medical syndromes then we would expect that with ongoing research, we would begin to see biological correlates that identify and separate them in a valid fashion. However, no such biological evidence has yet emerged, despite years of studies searching for reliable peripheral pathophysiological correlates in these conditions.

We believe it is important to keep an open mind about the possible underlying causes in any individual presenting with medically unexplained syndromes. In the instance of the conditions discussed above, it is still possible that further research may reveal specific pathological causes. Until then, we believe that the evidence is very persuasive that many (if not all) patients with these conditions are suffering from Somatoform Disorders. We feel it our duty to state that belief plainly, as it is important to offer these patients an understanding of their conditions, as this in turn can lead to effective management and substantial relief of suffering. The more accurately a diagnostic model reflects the underlying pathophysiology, the more effective will be the treatments based on that model.

We would strongly encourage clinicians to seriously consider the possibility of a primary somatoform process being causative in individuals with diagnoses such as Fibromyalgia, Chronic Fatigue Syndrome, and others mentioned above.

Somatoform Disorders may develop after relatively minor physical injuries

In the vast majority of individuals who sustain minor injuries to the head, neck, shoulders, back or limbs, there follows a natural course of recovery over a few days or weeks. A minority of such injuries, however, result in ongoing disability, in some cases a downward spiral to severe disruption of function, with symptoms and disability far out of proportion to that which one would expect from the initial injury. In clinical situations like these, clinicians should always do whatever they can to look for sinister underlying causes. Nerve root impingement, covert fractures, cartilage or ligament damage, inflammatory arthritis and other peripheral pathologies can all perpetuate pain after injury. In a subgroup of those with ongoing disability after injury, however, no evidence of any such peripheral pathology can be found.

There is no doubt that a somatoform process is an important perpetuating factor for a significant proportion of people suffering severe chronic disability after relatively minor injuries. A common pattern is that the initial and early pain and other consequences of the injury, often accompanied by emotions related to the trauma, act as a nidus for the development of a more complex set of symptoms. Pain in a region of the body may cause muscle bracing and atypical posture that then leads to more anatomically extensive discomfort. Pain can also interfere with sleep, and that, in turn, can lead to the beginning of neurochemical disturbances, especially in vulnerable individuals. Medications used to treat early symptoms, in particular opiates, may give short term relief (from both pain and dysphoria) but longitudinally may worsen overall function, causing symptoms such as fatigue. Emotions in response to the injury are particularly important. Some injuries are accompanied by intense fear and, in the worst case scenarios, a PTSD-type response. Other injuries may be accompanied by associated feelings of profound loss, shame, guilt, or intense anger and blame. The context of the injury is particularly important in this regard, and understandably shapes emotional response.

Somatoform reactions to injury are context dependent

Let us consider a variety of accidents leading to pain in a young boy that may have heuristic use when considering somatoform reactions to injury. Consider a relatively minor blow to the thigh that a child sustains under various circumstances and how the circumstances shape the child's response to that blow.

In the first instance, let us imagine a 7-year-old boy on the morning of his birthday running down the stairs in anticipation of a birthday gift. As he turns the corner on the stairs, he bumps his right thigh against the corner of the stairway, perhaps stumbles for a single step but in his excitement to get downstairs he essentially ignores the blow completely from then on. This blow has absolutely no consequences to his health or function.

For a second example, consider the same child who is now playing tag in the yard with his aunt. He is becoming tired of the game and slightly physically tired too. He bumps his thigh in a blow that is identical to the one described previously but on this occasion clutches his thigh, falls to the ground and complains to his aunt of the pain. This results in them discontinuing the game of tag, the child returns indoors. Shortly thereafter he begins to play a video game, which he enjoys, and which distracts him from the discomfort of the blow. He gives the blow to his leg no further thought thereafter and, indeed, experiences no further discomfort.

In the third example, that same child bumps his thigh in an identical fashion while running about his home on a Sunday where he is facing a week at school that is going to be somewhat distressing for him. He is not particularly enjoying one or two of his subjects, he has had a falling out with somebody he considered his best friend, there is something social going on at recess that makes school less attractive to him that week, and so on. On this occasion, he continues to experience discomfort in the thigh, complains of the pain to the point that his parents are worried enough to seek medical assistance for him the following day, which then results in him missing all of the next day's school and part of the following day's school for investigations. By mid-week sinister problems have been excluded and the boy returns to school. By the end of the week there is no further leg pain.

Now consider a fourth example, where the same child receives an identical blow but in this event it is intentionally caused by his brother during an altercation. Or a fifth example where the blow is the result of parental negligence or even physical abuse. Or a sixth example where along with receiving the blow himself, the boy caused more significant injuries to others. We could expect very different experiences of and reactions to such blows.

In each of the above scenarios, the actual blow to the body has been identical and has been sustained by the very same person, and in each case the natural history of the trivial peripheral injury could be expected to be straightforward, and to end with complete recovery. However, because of the very different contexts, the child's experience of and response to the blow has been quite different. These variations in response are unconscious and involuntary, the child actually experiences the blow in a different way depending on context, and in each case, responds according to that experience.

To now return to the broader subject of Somatoform Disorders that follow injuries, one can use the above exercise to encourage oneself to consider how context of injury can influence subsequent response and disability in any individual. When assessing response to injury, a careful analysis of accompanying emotions and attributions is essential.

These considerations can be particularly important when there are legal issues at play, where attempts to attribute blame for the consequences of injuries become issues of contention. Treatment of patients who are genuinely ill with a somatoform reaction to injury can be confounded by the fact that the patient may also stand to gain financially from ongoing disability. Even patients with the strongest desire to recover, and the very best intentions to not let legal considerations stand in the way of recovery, can be unconsciously hindered by these factors. These situations can present challenges for the treating clinician, who must attempt to understand the various factors at play and share that understanding with their patients as plainly as possible.

The common issue of suspected willful causation

1. Differentiating somatoform disorders from factitious disorder and malingering

There are no unequivocally reliable instruments for differentiating somatoform symptoms from symptoms that are consciously feigned, as may occur in factitious disorder or malingering. As you will see in the 'Assessment' section, there are many indicators that suggest that signs or symptoms may be psychogenic, but they do not reliably differentiate between conscious or unconscious cause. One will recall that the form of a somatoform symptom is driven by the patient's understanding of physiology and disease, and by the belief that they suffer from the presented physical symptoms. Thus both the malingerer and the somatoform sufferer are presenting a symptom determined by an idea, but the former knows they are acting while the latter believes that the idea reflects the truth.

The only way to differentiate these groups is by a thorough clinical assessment, and for the clinician to make a judgment regarding the veracity of the patient's apparent belief. The crucial question for the clinician to answer is thus:
"After very thorough assessment, do you, the clinician, believe that the patient believes that they are ill in this fashion?"
If the answer is "yes", then they have a Somatoform Disorder; if "no" there is a factitious or malingering component.

In most clinical settings, Somatoform Disorders are far more prevalent than factitious disorders or malingering. To make this issue even more complex, the line between these subdivisions is likely not razor sharp.

Very occasionally we have encountered a patient with a Somatoform Disorder where a chronic overall syndrome is clearly largely involuntary, but where there is evidence of some conscious exaggeration of one or two symptoms. Sometimes this is only a very small part of a very long duration illness, but the conclusion is still that there is a factitious component. This conscious amplification is, in these cases, perhaps performed to ensure that the severity of the illness is duly recognized by caregivers and clinicians. Ironically, it may come in a setting where the patient feels disbelieved. Such conscious feigning is dangerous because it can be interpreted as evidence that the entire condition is fabricated, and treatment and support consequently derailed or abandoned. Obviously, careful assessment of the entire picture is required.

> **Clinical Vignette:** *A 17-year-old woman with a lifelong history of spina bifida, right ankle dystonia, and bowel & bladder difficulties, was admitted to the inpatient neuropsychiatry unit after a prolonged chronic pain condition evolved into non-epileptic seizures and paraparesis. After comprehensive assessment, she was diagnosed with a Somatoform Disorder that seemed to be driven by underlying adjustment disorder with anxious & depressed mood. Treatment consisted of psychotherapy, physical therapies, and a psychotropic medication. A few days after commencing treatment, tablets were found in the waste-basket in her room, indicating conscious thwarting of the plan on the patient's part. Some members of the multidisciplinary treating team wondered if her entire presentation was factitious. However, exploration revealed this act to have been a manifestation of her ambivalence and tentativeness about her trust in the treating team, and about her faith in psychiatric treatment in general. Over a prolonged period of therapy she improved her coping skills, her psychiatric & physical symptoms, and her functioning. Although she still remains far behind her peers in emotional development, and despite this one episode of deliberately sabotaging her care, in the subsequent fifteen years she has been followed there has been no evidence of intentionally fabricated symptoms, and her presentation remains consistent with a Somatoform Disorder.*

2. Secondary gain is just that: 'secondary'

Patients with Somatoform Disorders will use their illnesses and sick role to gain whatever benefits they feel and believe may be their due. This is no different from how other individuals act with other illnesses, and should thus be an expected component of the clinical picture. When patients with Somatoform Disorders solicit support from relatives, or request special accommodations from the workplace, or claim insurance benefits that are their due, this is understandable. These 'benefits' of illness are labeled 'secondary gain'.

Secondary gains are less direct than the gain that is 'primary' - that of immediate reduction in emotional distress, which we understand to be the core engine that drives the illness.

When individuals with Somatoform Disorders seek secondary benefits, some onlookers, including in some instances their own medical caregivers or family members, may see this behaviour as evidence of some form of malingering. We do not see it as such, and we counsel clinicians and other caregivers to use a similar approach.

> **Clinical Vignette:** *A 29-year-old man experienced an increasing sense of physical fatigue, steadily worsening over months. Medical workup revealed no identifiable cause. He came to believe that the only way to overcome his fatigue was complete rest, so he took to bed. He involved himself in absolutely no activities except rest. He paid his roommate to empty a urinal that he kept by his bedside. He made one excursion a day out of his bedroom, to empty his bowels and to gather food from the refrigerator. He believed that this regimen resulted in periods of slow recovery, but improvements were inevitably thwarted by intrusions such as unexpected phone calls that then put him "back to square one". As a result, he remained completely disabled in this fashion for more than three years. He applied for and received the lowest level of government medical disability pension, barely enough to cover his very low expenses. During the process of assessment, some medical caregivers voiced the opinion that he may have been voluntarily behaving in this fashion, 'for secondary gain'.*

A question that can sometimes be helpful to consider, in this and other similar cases is: "Is it worth it?" For this individual, is this a 'good deal'? Is this 29-year-old man choosing to voluntarily confine himself to bed, in exchange for a meagre disability income and the convenience of having his urinal emptied by his roommate? Clearly, this is a very bad deal, to forgo a more active life for those 'benefits'. Obviously, one must consider the details from the perspective of the individual, as each of us value income and support to different degrees, and bring different psychological factors to bear on the equation. But as in the case above, more often than not 'secondary gain' is relatively paltry when considered against the effects of the illness, and is not the main driving engine behind the illness.

In our experience, most 'secondary gain' is simply the result of an individual with an illness attempting to make do as best as possible with that which is available to them. That said, in some cases, secondary benefits of illness and sick role may contribute to the perpetuation of illness, and this factor may need to be addressed specifically as part of the management plan.

The neurobiology of somatization will prove to be very complex

The pathophysiology of Somatoform Disorders will eventually be described at the tissue and molecular level, and we can be sure that it will be shown to be very complex. Consider that the manifestation of a somatoform symptom may involve neural systems responsible for emotion, cognition (including belief and insight), perception, and movement. Some or all of these neural components would be expected to function atypically in a Somatoform Disorder. Thus, to identify, dissect, and fully understand the neurobiology of somatoform syndromes is going to be a very complex task. This is particularly daunting given that we don't yet have a comprehensive neurobiological understanding of most of the separate components. Furthermore, there may be more than one single pathway by which somatoform symptoms are produced.

At some time in the future we would expect that these conditions will be understood at the molecular level, but it is unlikely that any imminent neurobiological advances will change our approach to the understanding and management of these conditions in the near future.

There may prove to be some valid subdivisions of somatoform symptoms reflecting differences in underlying pathogenesis

As these disorders are better understood and better classified, there will likely emerge some valid subdivisions. For instance, somatoform conditions resulting from underlying anxiety will likely be more prone to emerge as physical conditions that represent an exaggeration or misinterpretation of the direct physiological effects of anxiety.

It is also possible that there may prove to be subgroups of individuals presenting with somatoform symptoms or signs that are caused by dysregulation of very specific relevant brain circuitry. For example, consider that there may be a highly preserved mammalian reflex to retract an injured limb, leading a limb to appear 'paralyzed' without gross neurological cause.

There is work that is currently exploring the possibilities of specific neurobiological underpinnings to somatoform syndromes, and at some point this may lead to very specific treatment options for some subgroups. This work is preliminary, however, and investigative techniques do not yet allow us to identify, nor treat, subgroups of individuals in any specifically beneficial fashion. Until any valid subdivisions are identified in a clinically useful manner, we recommend using the approach described in this book, which involves customizing an understanding of the emotional distress and physical symptoms for each individual patient. Nothing is lost clinically with this approach. Until we can 'lump' in a valid fashion, we should be thorough and reductionistic when it comes to attempting to dissect and understand each patient's physical symptoms, and the nature of their own specific underlying emotional distress. This approach works best clinically, and is also more likely to ultimately facilitate advances in our understanding of the underlying neurobiology.

References:

Aaron LA, Buchwald D: A review of the evidence for overlap among unexplained clinical conditions. Ann Intern Med 2001; 134:868-81

Aggarwal VR, McBeth J, Zakrzewska JM, Lunt M, Macfarlane GJ. The epidemiology of chronic syndromes that are frequently unexplained: do they have common associated factors? Int J Epidemiol 2006; 35:468–76

Delis D, Witter S: Cogniform Disorder and Cogniform Condition: Proposed diagnoses for excessive cognitive symptoms. Archives of Clinical Neuropsychology 2007; 22:589-604

De Waal MW, Arnold IA, Eekhof JA, van Hemert AM: Somatoform disorders in general practice: prevalence, functional impairment and comorbidity with anxiety and depressive disorders. British Journal of Psychiatry 2004; 184:470-6

Fink P, Sørensen L, Engberg M, Holm M, Munk-Jørgensen P: Somatization in primary care. Prevalence, health care utilization, and general practitioner recognition. Psychosomatics 1999; 40:330-8

Kirmayer LJ, Young A: Culture and somatization: clinical, epidemiological, and ethnographic perspectives. Psychosom Med 1998; 60:420-30

Mattila AK, Kronholm E, Jula A, Salminen JK, Koivisto AM, Mielonen RL, Joukamaa M: Alexithymia and somatization in general population. Psychosom Med 2008; 70:716-22

Schur EA, Afari N, Furberg H, Olarte M, Goldberg J, Sullivan PF, Buchwald D. Feeling bad in more ways than one: comorbidity patterns of medically unexplained and psychiatric conditions. J Gen Intern Med 2007; 22:818–21

Simeon D, Smith RJ, Knutelska M, Smith LM: Somatoform dissociation in depersonalization disorder. J Trauma Dissociation 2008; 9:335-48

Snijders TJ, de Leeuw FE, Klumpers UM, Kappelle LJ, van Gijn J: Prevalence and predictors of unexplained neurological symptoms in an academic neurology outpatient clinic--an observational study. J Neurol 2004; 251:66-71

Spiers-Lopez, P: 'Executive Life: The Boss; It's Show Time'. The New York Times, 7 March 2004

Stone J, Carson A, Duncan R, Coleman R, Roberts R, Warlow C, Hibberd C, Murray G, Cull R, Pelosi A, Cavanagh J, Matthews K, Goldbeck R, Smyth R, Walker J, Macmahon AD, Sharpe M: Symptoms 'unexplained by organic disease' in 1144 new neurology out-patients: how often does the diagnosis change at follow-up? Brain 2009; 132: 2878–88

Wald J, Taylor S, Scamvougeras A: Cognitive Behavioural and Neuropsychiatric treatment of post-traumatic Conversion Disorder: a case study. Cognitive Behaviour Therapy 2004; 33:12–20

Wessely S, Nimnuan C, Sharpe M: Functional somatic syndromes: one or many? Lancet 1999; 354:936-9

CHAPTER 3

REFERRAL

Case detection

Ideally, we would be able to identify each and every individual with a Somatoform Disorder who could benefit from available treatments. These syndromes, however, particularly mild forms, have a natural tendency to hide themselves, a result of the patient being unconscious of the nature of the condition and of clinicians preferring to interpret them as physical concerns. Despite this, they come to light in different ways and in different settings. A family practitioner may notice a pattern of unusual or difficult to explain symptoms & signs in a regular patient; a neurologist may note signs that are unequivocally 'functional'; a physiotherapist may observe an unusual pattern of limb movement or gait; a gastroenterologist may note an atypical pattern of pain or disproportionate disability; a psychiatrist may note a great deal of changeable physical symptoms in a patient referred for emotional distress. Most experienced primary care physicians will be aware that they have in their practice a small number of patients with particularly challenging chronic somatoform syndromes.

Being faced with a patient with medically unexplained symptoms can be unsettling and confusing for many clinicians, many of whom do not have a framework around which to understand them, nor a straightforward approach to management. General clinicians are often uncomfortable to infer a psychiatric diagnosis, or may present this possibility to the patient in a manner that the patient finds difficult to accept. Patients may be reluctant to agree to a psychiatric assessment or may consider it unnecessary.

Psychiatrists who do have an opportunity to assess these patients may feel uncomfortable with the primarily physical nature of the presentation, or with the task of confirming somatization in the absence of overt psychiatric co-morbidity. Referrals to general psychiatrists in cases of suspected Somatoform Disorder may be declined on account of a lack of the psychiatrist's experience or interest, or due to an arbitrary decision that the patient may not meet a threshold of manifest psychopathology. Some mental health centres may only treat patients with clearly identifiable, persistent and severe diagnosed mental conditions such as Bipolar Affective Disorder or Schizophrenia, and systematically decline patients with somatoform presentations.

In most modern clinical settings there is a need for a clear approach to assessing patients who are suspected of suffering Somatoform Disorders, or alternatively, for clearly identified local experts or teams to whom such patients can be referred.

Who should assess and treat?

The majority of cases of Somatoform Disorder are mild in severity and will improve with examination, investigations, and/or reassurance with some psychological need being met, or the inciting stressor resolving, or the attenuation of a temporary disturbance in mental function. Many likely resolve without being identified as somatoform in nature.

Patients with moderate somatization will probably require more active input from the family physician, the non-psychiatric specialists for reassurance regarding the absence of organic disease, and a psychiatrist or psychologist who can actively manage their psychiatric symptoms and help the patient understand and resolve psychological distress.

Patients with severe somatization will likely require ongoing management by the family doctor, the treating psychiatrist, and a sub-specialist referral to psychiatrists and/or psychologists with expertise in assessing and treating Somatoform Disorders. Sometimes multidisciplinary team and/or inpatient treatment is required.

Ideally, dedicated multidisciplinary teams with members that include general physicians, psychiatrists, non-psychiatric specialists, nurses, occupational & physical therapists, and psychologists would be available to patients as required, but this is rarely the case. The need for dedicated multidisciplinary outpatient clinics cannot be understated, particularly for those suffering severe forms of the disorder. Such clinics would greatly improve the quality of care that most individuals suffering these disorders are currently receiving.

Resources the treating clinicians will require

Adequate time is a necessity, as a thorough assessment on an outpatient basis will require a series of consecutive visits, and management includes regular and at times frequent follow-up. The clinician needs to be able to offer longitudinal care. Method of remuneration is a practical and important consideration. A health care system that offers the clinician remuneration for time spent is perhaps essential. This factor alone often determines that psychiatrists may be in a better position to offer treatment, especially when compared with family practitioners, or specialists such as psychologists, internists or neurologists, who may not work under a structure that offers fair remuneration for the necessary time spent.

Adequate skills are required for ascertaining the atypical presentation of physical symptoms and signs, in eliciting psychiatric complaints, in developing an understanding of the person's emotional distress & coping mechanisms, and in managing the disorder using psychotherapy, pharmacotherapy and/or physical therapies. These skills may all be developed by individual clinicians, or more commonly, shared amongst members of the team assessing and treating the patient. Clinicians competent in the psychopharmacological management of psychiatric conditions, in cognitive behavioural therapy and interpersonal therapy, and in physical therapies should be available in the management stages. Ideally, physical therapies will be conducted by physiotherapists, or in some cases occupational therapists, who have experience treating patients with severe and persistent functional physical symptoms. Patients may initially be averse to, or misunderstand, the therapeutic value of physical therapies and behavioural activation, and the clinicians providing those interventions should ideally be able to put these therapies into context.

A certain degree of psychotherapeutic skill is paramount. The patient most needs the clinician to recognize their suffering as emotional, to assess the possible causes of their emotional distress as carefully as possible, and to then work using interventions designed to decrease that suffering. The type of psychotherapeutic work will vary from clinician to clinician, depending on their preferred approach. A good therapeutic alliance greatly increases the chances of a positive outcome.

Work with Somatoform Disorder patients can be very challenging, but at the same time professionally gratifying. Clinicians may ask themselves if they have the adequate desire, patience, and tenacity to be treating patients with more severe forms of these disorders. Patients may feel blamed, defensive, guilty, angry, and misunderstood. Some patients will be convinced they are physically ill, and sometimes those beliefs are held with delusional intensity. The capacity for the treating clinician to understand and tolerate counter-transference is essential. Does the clinician believe they can help the patient? Do they see patients with somatization as legitimately being in need? Can they manage episodes of perceived empathic failure or being blamed for treatment failures? Do they themselves have an adequately supportive framework such that they are able to offer care that may present significant challenges? Does the clinician have sufficient back-up or support in the event that the patient experiences overwhelming emotional distress or in the event that overt and difficult to treat psychopathology emerges (as sometimes occurs when somatization defences retreat)?

A common scenario

In a busy general practice, a patient seems to be suffering the effects of somatization. They complain of chronic intractable physical symptoms, the majority of which have been inadequately explained despite adequate assessment and investigations. The patient has repeatedly presented for medical attention. They are functionally disabled, despite support being provided. Yet no definitive diagnosis has been made and no clear management plan is in place. The clinician, the patient, and their support network are all frustrated by the lack of progress. The patient is referred for assessment to a clinician who works to help individuals with somatoform presentations.

CHAPTER 4

ASSESSMENT

Assessment of a Patient with Suspected Somatoform Disorder

Having been referred a patient with a suspected Somatoform Disorder, the clinician's initial task is to perform a thorough assessment. The first step in doing so is to genuinely open one's mind to the possibility that the individual is *not* suffering from somatization. The assessment must not automatically confirm the referral source's suspicion of psychogenesis.

Initiate the therapeutic alliance

The assessment begins with first contact. The most important task at this point is to initiate a sound therapeutic alliance.

Even at that early stage, the clinician will know enough to be able to genuinely declare that the individual is clearly suffering from a serious condition, which is markedly impairing his or her quality of life. Patients later report that this validation is an extremely encouraging aspect of the assessment.

One should express the expectation that the assessment will allow for a thorough understanding of the disorder, and that management options will subsequently be proposed.

Set up the framework for the assessment

The process and purpose of the assessment are explained in advance. It is best to outline that the assessment will require a historical review of the emotional and physical context in which the symptoms developed, a careful and comprehensive understanding of the symptoms over time including their current status, discussion about the past history of similar symptoms, as well as of the person's past health concerns, and their physical and emotional development. Explain that the purpose of this is to thoroughly understand the symptoms in order to determine their cause. This will be assisted by a physical examination by the clinician or a suitable specialist, and a screen of intellectual functions. The need for further information from collateral sources should be discussed. It should be stated that all previous investigations and trials of therapies and other interventions will be reviewed. The patient should be invited to raise any pressing questions before the formal history begins, and any questions or concerns about the nature of the assessment should be addressed. The patient's expectations and intentions are therefore laid out and explored in advance.

Be clear regarding phases of process

It is helpful to keep clear in one's own mind the three distinct clinical phases, namely: assessment, formulation and management. It is particularly important to delay formulation and to resist any temptation to make major alterations in management until after assessment. One does not want to share opinions or change treatments based on incomplete information. The assessment phase should focus almost entirely on gathering data and attempting to understand the patient's predicament. The rationale for obtaining a thorough understanding prior to implementing interventions should be communicated to the patient prior to commencing: we cannot treat effectively until we are clear about diagnosis. For the vast majority of patients this is reassuring but at the same time difficult, as they may be presenting with pressing or even urgent symptoms.

Avoid premature closure

When assessing an individual with a probable severe Somatoform Disorder, it is of paramount importance that treating clinicians not arrive at premature conclusions regarding diagnosis. This is particularly challenging when patients are referred with a presumed Somatoform Disorder diagnosis and there already exists substantial documentation of prior inconclusive consultations and investigations. Although one must obviously make use of such information, the clinician is advised that his or her own assessment process should be as comprehensive as possible. A brief assessment and opinion is highly unlikely to contribute to the understanding of the problem, and will likely be perceived as superficial or dismissive by the patient. Patients commonly expect to be disbelieved. They are anticipating that clinicians will approach them with skepticism. They will often make statements such as: "I was told this was not a real illness" or "they said it is all in my head." It almost goes without saying that it is important for the clinician to thoroughly understand that the patient is genuinely incapacitated, and to consequently adopt an empathic and non-judgmental position throughout.

History-taking must be thorough, and as a result is time-intensive

A comprehensive assessment is infinitely superior to a cursory one, which is arguably of very little value. A brief one-session assessment of a patient with a complex disorder most often turns out to be little more than a 'reconnaissance flight.' If the condition is more severe and more chronic, the patient has likely had many such assessments through the course of their illness, and another such cursory assessment will likely make little difference.

The thorough assessment aims to gather as much data as possible about the patient and his or her condition, such that a definitive diagnosis can be reached, and such that it is clear to the patient that all aspects of the illness have been considered.

The clinician should allow the patient to describe their symptoms in as much detail as is necessary. Any attempt to hurry this process will likely be interpreted by the patient as disregard, and may render the entire assessment effectively useless.

The initial assessment session will usually be used to get an introduction to the patient's current psychosocial situation and functioning, and to exhaustively review each current disabling symptom. Attention is paid to the onset, course, nature, severity, and exacerbating & alleviating factors for each symptom. This review will often alert the clinician to atypical aspects of the presenting symptoms.

It will commonly take three or four hours to complete an assessment, sometimes considerably more. Reviewing records and obtaining history from collateral sources, including family and other treating clinicians, may also require a considerable amount of time and effort. The assessing clinician should be working within a framework that supports this use of their time. The time is well invested as it lays the foundation for potentially successful management, and allows a therapeutic alliance to develop. If it had been present, a patient's initial guardedness and irritability often settles through the process of a careful and methodical assessment.

Psychiatric History and Mental Status Examination

Ensure that a comprehensive psychiatric assessment is performed, as it would be for any other patient.

The psychiatric components of assessment include: the exploration of psychosocial or biological antecedents to the presenting illness episode; the past psychiatric, family, developmental and relationship history; a screen for current psychiatric symptoms; and a mental status examination, including bedside testing of higher cognitive-intellectual functions (aspects of which are considered along with the neurological examination later in this chapter).

The psychiatric examination allows for identification of any overt major psychiatric syndromes as well as psychological themes and conflicts. It explores the level of functioning the individual has demonstrated over the course of their life, and may give some idea of the nature of their defences (including the tendency to avoid challenging emotional states). It also may uncover any prominent sources of emotional distress at the time of the onset of the condition.

It is particularly important to thoroughly explore neurovegetative features such as sleep, energy, libido, appetite and weight, as any disturbance in these realms may be evidence of gross neurobiological dysfunction and clues to underlying Axis I psychiatric conditions. Neurovegetative changes may exist without obvious emotional changes, sometimes because no such emotional change exists, but in other cases because the emotional change is largely hidden, in much the same way as this can occur in alexithymic individuals who are unable to directly express emotional distress.

An additional important element in history-taking in the somatizing patient is to explore for a past history of unexplained physical symptoms. On account of the retrospective nature of this self-assessment, it is fraught with error. However, a past history of frequent visits to medical caregivers for unclear reasons, or of diagnoses of functional somatic syndromes such as Chronic Fatigue Syndrome, Fibromyalgia, or Irritable Bowel Syndrome, is important for one's understanding.

An initial screening question may alert the clinician to the need for further exploration: "Have you in the past struggled for long periods of time with bothersome physical symptoms for which the underlying cause could not be found?"

Assess the patient's attribution theories

It is important to understand the patient's own understanding of their condition. Why do they think they are unwell in this fashion? What mechanisms do they believe are underlying their symptoms? This information is useful when one is looking for a heuristic model on which to base treatment. The clinician should seek common ground between their own ideas and the patient's way of conceptualizing the illness.

Exploring attributions emphasizes to the patient that their experience of the illness is central, and that the finer points of their own understanding of the symptoms are seen as important. Assessing the patient's attribution theories also allows the clinician to assess for uncertainty in the patient's understanding, or for a cognitive inflexibility that may denote a defensiveness towards a psychiatric interpretation of the cause of the suffering. Atypical fixed beliefs or bizarre ideas may suggest somatic delusions.

It is at times tempting to correct the individual's attributions during the assessment phase, particularly if the explanations are clearly not biologically plausible. However, doing so prior to the end of the assessement and before formulation will likely be perceived as dismissive. It is best for the clinician to remain objective, uncertain, and inquisitive, and to put effort into trying to understand how misconceptions developed.

Illustration 1:

Drawing & text spontaneously created by a patient with a Somatoform Disorder to relay severity and nature of their symptoms to their assessing clinician

Note the descriptions and breadth of their disabilities: along with many physical symptoms, their "taste, hobbies, humour, creativity, stamina, abilities" are affected. "Everything" is "off".

Published here with specific permission from the patient.

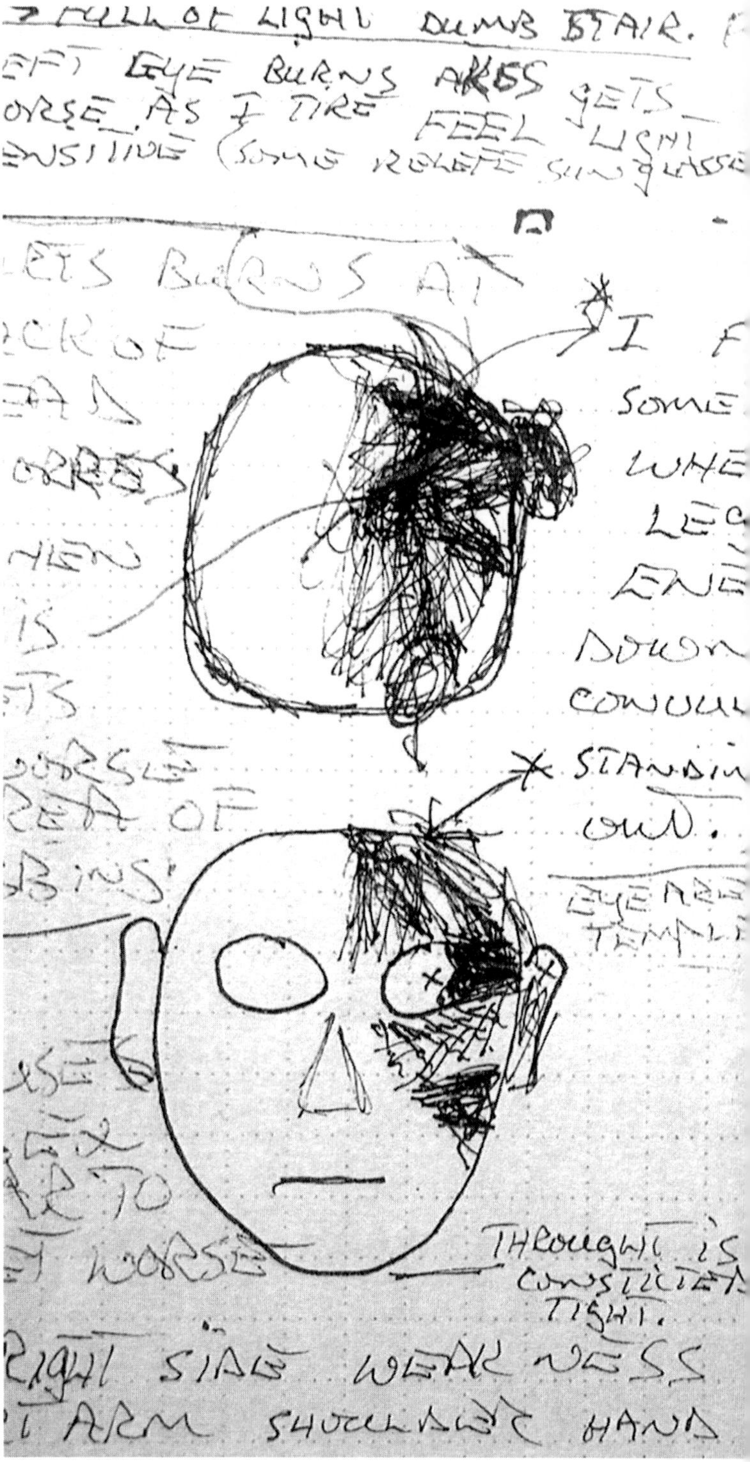

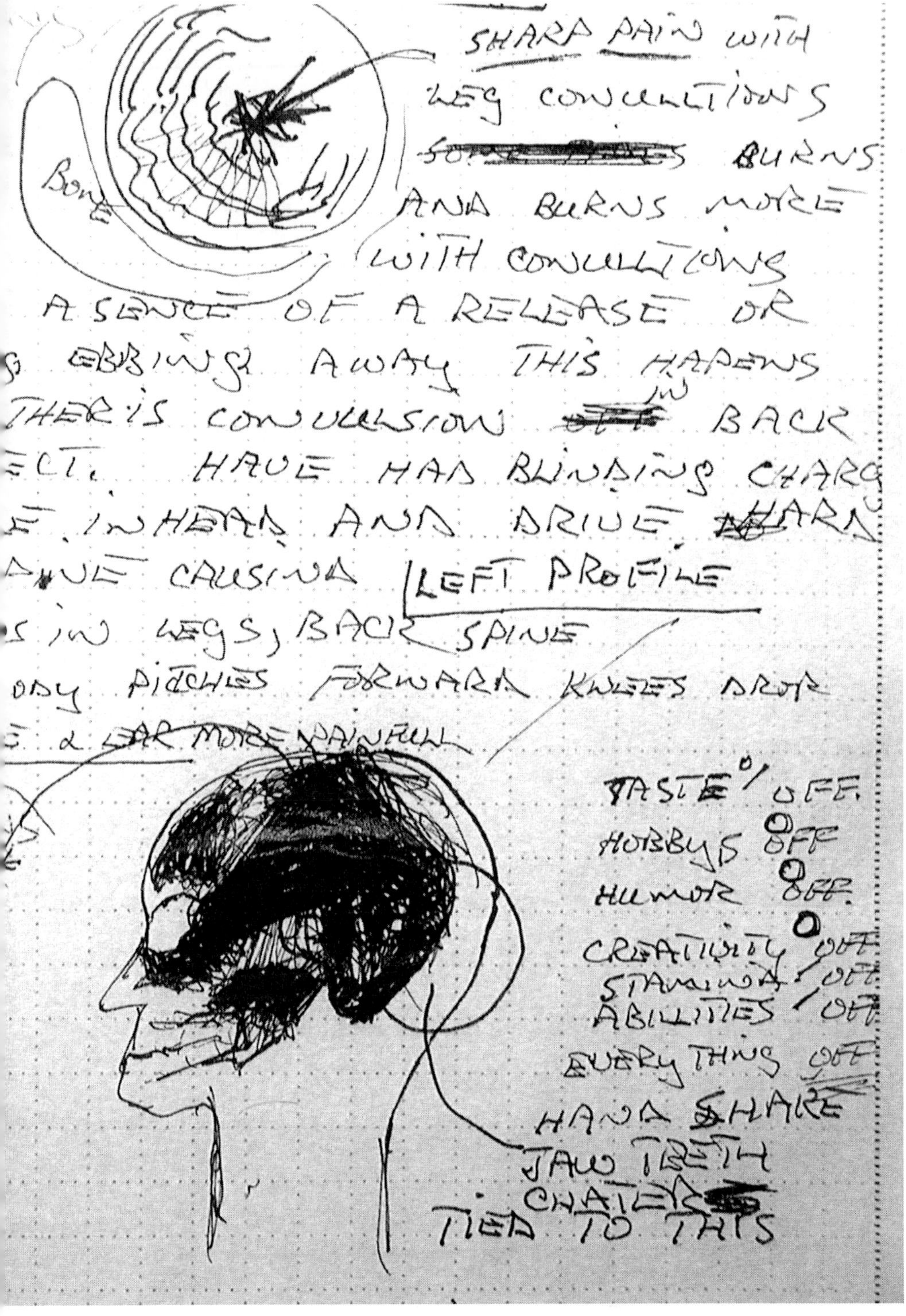
Bone
SHARP PAIN WITH
LEG CONVULLTIONS
BURNS
AND BURNS MORE
WITH CONVULLTIONS
A SENCE OF A RELEASE OR
EBBING AWAY THIS HAPENS
THERE IS CONVULSION IN BACK
ECT. HAVE HAD BLINDING CHARG
E IN HEAD AND DRIVE HARD
DIVE CAUSING
LEFT PROFILE
S IN LEGS, BACK SPINE
ODY PITCHES FORWARD KNEES DROP
E & EAR MORE PAINFUL
TASTE 0/OFF
HOBBYS 0 OFF
HUMOR 0 OFF
CREATIVITY 0/OFF
STAMINA /OFF
ABILITIES /OFF
EVERYTHING OFF
HAND SHAKE
JAW TEETH
CHATTERS
TIED TO THIS

Listen to the patient's language

Listen carefully to how the patient describes their symptoms and signs, and what phrases they use to attempt to explain underlying mechanisms. Language use is a clue to attributions, and patient labels for central aspects of their disorder can later be useful when it comes to describing a cognitive framework for understanding their condition, and for guiding therapy.

> **Clinical Vignette:** *A 41-year-old former dancer, twenty years prior to presentation, suffered from a flu-like illness with subsequent debilitating fatigue. She had been on self-imposed bed-rest for thirteen years before seeking a psychiatric opinion. She referred to her limited energy as her "reserve," and believed that for every quantum of energy she expended, she required rest to "recover." After a formulation was presented to her in emotional rather than physical terms, the use of the metaphor of emotional "recovery" from stressful situations and events continued to be used and helped her improve her functioning.*

Medical History and Systems Review

Perform a careful review of past medical problems. Do a comprehensive review of systems in order to look for symptoms that may not initially be volunteered as presenting concerns, whether disease-based or somatoform. This will decrease the chances of unexpected symptom substitution in the future when an alternate symptom may manifest as a result of the same underlying threat or emotional state. During assessment one wants to attempt to comprehend *all* of the somatoform symptoms and signs, so that as the treatment proceeds they can be dealt with together even as each is kept individually in mind.

Physical Examination of the Somatoform patient

Somatoform Disorders are clinical diagnoses. While ancillary tests may reassure both the clinician and the patient that a disease does not appear responsible for the patient's presentation, a thorough and careful physical examination is central to the assessment.

Traditionally, clinicians have sought to eliminate evidence of disease by examining the patient and reaching the diagnosis of somatization by excluding non-psychiatric medical disorders. A normal neurological examination, while reassuring, is nonspecific, and is by itself nonconfirmatory. Despite physical examination features that are commonly seen in these conditions, there are no absolute pathognomonic signs of conversion or other Somatoform Disorders. Inter-rater reliability and test-retest reliability of the vast majority of physical signs of Somatoform Disorders (including conversion disorder and somatoform pain disorder) are limited. False positive signs may occur due to unrelated variables such as pain, neglect, or inattention, and thus do not necessarily indicate psychogenicity. One must take into account various clues from the history and examination to make a confident diagnosis.

The hallmark of the examination of the somatoform patient is the discovery of a *multitude* of abnormalities that cannot be explained by our understanding of neuroanatomy, neuropathology and the usual pathophysiology of neurological and non-neurological diseases. One must be vigilant for atypical presentations. Hence, the approach to the physical examination is an individualized and customized endeavour.

Certain 'positive signs' of somatization have long been described. These clinical markers, rather than representing the absence of something, represent definite evidence that a psychogenic process is creating a symptom or sign. The descriptions below summarize some of the classic psychogenic findings with prominent focus on the neurological exam:

General observation and examination

Upon observing the patient put on or remove his or her shoes or jacket, manipulate objects, walk into the room or into the building, one may note inexplicable inconsistencies when compared to how they are able to move when they are on the examining table. Pain and other abnormal illness behaviours such as wincing, anticipatory withdrawal, lying down, repeated standing and walking, or holding the affected area should be noted. The patient may ask to have the lights off or voluntarily close their eyes during the interview or may sigh excessively.

Speech may be excessively slow with a long latency. Stutter may occur in the middle but not at the end of sentences, may worsen with emotionally distressing content, or may be noted to be interrupted by perfectly articulated sounds. Word-finding difficulties may be noted, and speech may become telegrammatic, with inclusion of only nouns and verbs.

Measurement of vital signs may yield nonspecific hypertension and/or tachycardia. Diaphoresis may be noted as well as other signs of autonomic excitability. Atypical and inconsistent breathing patterns should be documented.

Atypical findings on examination of the head and neck, respiratory, cardiovascular, urogenital, endocrinological, and dermatological systems should be documented. These systems are examined to look for the presence of signs of general medical illnesses.

On examination of the gastrointestinal system, bloating of the abdomen may reflect air on percussion which does not shift with position and is relieved with sedation.

Musculoskeletal examination may reveal multiple tender points, in the absence of inflammatory changes and muscle wasting, and may include Fibromyalgia "trigger points" (the anterior aspects of the C5 and C7 intertransverse spaces, the upper border of the mid-portion of the trapezii, the insertion of the nuchal muscles at the occiput, the muscle attachments to the upper medial border of the scapula, the second rib space lateral to the sternal border, the attachments of the lateral epicondyle and the greater trochanter, the medial fat pad adjacent to the joint line of the knee, and the upper outer quadrant of the gluteal muscles). Typically, tender points are not limited to these areas.

Cognitive-intellectual examination

Variability of attentional function and motivation is common. Ganser-type (or 'near miss') responses may be evident. Performance on recognition memory tasks that falls below the likelihood of chance may be seen. Inconsistent responses may occur (e.g. the capacity to spell 5 or 6 letter words backwards accompanied by a backwards digit span of only 2 or 3).

Cranial nerve examination

A pseudo-anosmic patient fails to recognize the smell of alcohol which if adequately potent should stimulate nociceptors not osmoreceptors.

A patient reporting loss of visual acuity fails to recognize changes in stimulus luminosity in the peripheral field (preserved even in patients with optic atrophy).

Intermittent blurry vision or asthenopia may be produced by excessive peri-orbital muscular contraction and may be relieved by contraction and subsequent relaxation of these muscles.

A patient with pseudoptosis may demonstrate contraction of the orbicularis oculi and lessened activity of the frontalis muscle. Lateral gaze limitations are found to be due to convergence hyperactivity as seen by associated miosis.

Vibration sensation is split across the frontalis bone with the patient reporting diminished or absent sensation on the affected side. Facial sensory loss is reported to inconsistent stimuli (e.g. increased sensation of temperature with loss of sensation to pin) or in a nondermatomal pattern.

Weakness of the lower face is found to be due to orbicularis oris hyperactivity.

Deafness is reported despite preserved startle. Mutism is accompanied by preserved phonation on coughing and occurs in the absence of language disturbance, comprehension deficits, or reading and writing impairments.

Sternocleidomastoid weakness is noted despite a known bilateral innervation.

The tongue is deviated even at rest in the mouth and when protruded points to the unaffected side (due to excessive contraction of the affected side) not to the affected side due to ipsilateral muscle paresis (the last in disease affecting the hypoglossal nerve).

Motor examination

On strength testing, the patient is able to contract a muscle in one position but unable to contract the same muscle in another position. This variability may be more specific in certain situations. For example, when the patient is asked to contract the unaffected hip flexor while supine, the affected hip extensor reflexively contracts by evidence of downward pressure at the affected heel much more so than when the patient is asked to voluntarily extend the affected hip (Hoover sign). The Reverse Hoover sign is a lack of reflex extension of the unaffected hip with attempted flexion of the affected hip. Similarly shoulder abduction and adduction and hip abduction and adduction of the paretic limb may occur reflexively (and more so than with voluntary effort) with abduction and adduction of the unaffected limb.

Typically, a contraction of the antagonist muscle occurs before or simultaneous to contraction of the muscle the patient is asked to contract. Alternatively, full contraction is brief and followed quickly by relaxation, or normal strength is produced with marked variability in force such that effort appears stuttering or incomplete (referred to at times as "give-way weakness"). Typical pyramidal weakness is not observed, so that, for instance, plantar flexion appears more compromised than dorsiflexion at the ankle.

Tone may be characteristically paratonic, with apparent rigidity (regardless of direction or velocity of movement) that can be overcome. Tone may also attenuate with performance of simultaneous movements of the contralateral limb (this typically worsens rigidity in parkinsonism).

Reflexes are hyperactive although symmetrical. Plantar responses are mute or flexor, and inconsistent with the degree of weakness or increased tone.

Bulk is preserved. Sleep, sedation, or anaesthesia reveal that any perceived hypertrophy is reversible.

If involuntary movements are present, tremor may vary in amplitude, direction, or frequency. The tremor can be entrained to a different frequency when the patient focuses on a complex rhythmic movement of another body part. The tremor occurs both during movement and rest. Paroxysmal movements are elicited by unusual stimuli (e.g. certain sounds or words; vibration). Irregular movements can be attenuated by distraction (note that tics, stereotypies, and tardive akathisia can respond similarly) or may occur only with selective tasks. Excessive bradykinesia or bizarre movements may be present. A variety of abnormal movements (e.g. tremor, myoclonus, and gait disturbance) may co-occur. Parkinsonism may occur in the absence of fatiguing with decremental amplitude and arrest during ongoing movement. Parkinsonism is unaccompanied by hypomimia, axial rigidity, or decreased blink.

Paroxysmal events or attacks, such as non-epileptic seizures, may occur during the examination and may be precipitated by emotion. The spells may be accompanied by vocalizations, with maintenance of consciousness, bilateral flailing, head rotation movements, eye closure, asynchronous or tonic movements or, if tonic-clonic, without simultaneous back/abdominal muscle contraction (causing opisthotonus). There is an absence of typical epileptiform features such as tongue biting, extensor plantar responses, and abnormal pupillary reactions. The spells are often variable in the sequence of physical signs (rather than stereotyped) and prolonged in duration.

Sensory examination

On testing of cortical sensory signs, visual field deficits remain static regardless of the distance from the focal target. Peripheral vision is graded as perceived or not and not based on the intensity, nature or movement of the stimulus.

Exaggerated inattention or 'la belle indifference' may be evident towards the deficit in the absence of neglect or agnosia. Functional hemianopia is (typically) present with both eyes open but the field may be revealed in the unaffected eye with the affected eye closed.

On testing of specific sensory modalities, hypoaesthesia to all sensory modalities in sharply demarcated boundaries is common; during the perceived absence of position sense of a limb or digit, ask for the unaffected finger or limb to touch the affected part (this is absent in disease affecting proprioception due to complete loss of position sense whereas somatoform patients operate as if the intact position sense of the healthy part means it can find the affected part). Diminished ticklishness of the affected side has been reported.

In terms of the pattern of sensory deficits, perceived hypoaesthesia does not respect dermatomal or peripheral nerve distribution (e.g. patchy distribution, stocking and glove, cheek without buccal mucosa, abdomen without back, face exclusive of cornea or lips). There may be perceived loss of sensation (e.g. at the midline) to vibration that clearly passes from areas of preserved sensation (e.g. frontal bone or sternum). There are changing patterns of hypoaesthesia. Hemianaesthesia may precisely split the midline (sensory loss if not thalamic should be paramedian due to overlap of cutaneous branches of the intercostal nerves). The Bowlus maneuver, where the patient is asked to interlock their fingers with their arms crossed at the wrist, can reveal inconsistencies in altered sensation or movement.

If pain is present, it may be elicited by light touch (e.g. allodynia). Sensory modalities are not dissociated, if there is numbness to touch, there is reduced response to all modalities.

Waddell described eight signs in five categories thought to be indicative of a psychological component to pain, in particular, lower back pain. These include: tenderness (allodynia, nonanatomic deep tenderness not localized to one area); simulation (low back pain with axial loading on the skull, pain induced by shoulder and pelvic rotation); distraction (difference in straight leg raising in supine and sitting position); regional ("give-way" weakness in multiple muscle groups, nondermatomal sensory loss), and overreaction (disproportionate facial or verbal expressions to pain). Waddell's signs are more prognostic than diagnostic; their presence on examination (of at least three categories) can predict poor outcome in chronic pain patients (Waddell 1980).

Coordination, station, and gait testing

Functional patients may deviate more from touching the perceived target with the affected limb as the target is brought closer (it is the opposite pattern in cerebellar lesions). The patient perceives the affected leg as mildly weak when standing but may fall when asked to kick the affected leg despite standing on the unaffected leg or when asked to kick the unaffected leg maintains stance on the affected leg.

Romberg testing is positive but there is no swaying when the patient's eyes are incidentally covered by the examiner. Excessive sway on Romberg testing may actually demonstrate intact position sense.

An exaggerated response on push-pull test may be evident. Astasia abasia, the inability to stand or walk in a normal manner, may be elicited specifically by movements that cannot be completed while upright but are preserved while the patient is supine or sitting. Gait does not follow the normal pattern of disease (e.g. during monoplegic or hemiplegic gait, no circumduction of the hip is seen but rather the leg is dragged with the leg in external or internal rotation and the foot inverted or everted or pointing inwards or outwards). Gait may be markedly slow, 'uneconomic' (wasting muscle energy) or hesitant. Patients may appear to be 'walking on ice'. Knees may buckle without inducing a fall. A vertical shaking tremor may occur.

In summary, a thorough physical examination may be highly revealing of a somatoform diagnosis but only in the presence of a multitude of findings and when historical details are also considered. Findings on examination should be sought as rigorously in Somatoform Disorders as they are in organic conditions and clinicians should not be reassured solely by a normal examination.

Who should perform the physical examination?

Some psychiatrists working with patients with Somatoform Disorders may choose to request that the patient's family practitioner or an independent clinician perform the physical examination. If this is the case, close communication is necessary between the physicians.

There are considerable advantages to having the treating psychiatrist perform the physical examination:

-- It generally enhances rather than detracts from the therapeutic alliance.

-- It gives the psychiatrist a far more precise and first-hand understanding of each physical symptom and sign. This is particularly useful when it comes to formulating an understanding of the illness with the patient.

-- Having a literally 'hands-on' knowledge of the clinical signs adds credibility to the clinician's opinion when it comes to sharing a diagnosis. It carries far more weight when discussing a symptom when one has

closely examined the affected part of the body oneself.
-- It also serves to far more efficiently deal with any new symptoms once management has commenced: rather than initiating another string of referrals and wait-time delays, the psychiatrist who is comfortable with physical examination can often deal with new concerns immediately.

Having said all this, there is still an important place for referral to specialist colleagues to clarify or diagnose any physical findings that may be out of the ordinary, or suggestive of non-psychiatric illness.

Using the opinions of specialist colleagues to supplement one's own understanding of the patient's condition, however, doesn't make it any less beneficial to also perform the initial physical examination oneself.

There is also a place for requesting that the physical examination be conducted by an appropriate colleague if a more complex therapeutic relationship has already developed between the primary treating physician and the patient. The nature of the patient's transference and the type of psychological work that may have commenced, may make physical examination by the treating psychiatrist inappropriate later in the course of the therapy.

Special Investigations

Special investigations are conducted, as indicated by the clinical findings, to exclude conditions that may be causing the physical symptoms. It is also important to exclude general medical conditions that could be causing psychiatric symptoms that are subsequently masquerading as nonspecific physical symptoms. Conditions such as hypothyroidism, hyperthyroidism, abnormalities of calcium metabolism, Wilson's disease, early Huntington disease, ALS, dementia, other neurodegenerative conditions, seizure disorders, multiple sclerosis, malignancy, lupus and the autoimmune conditions, just to name a few, should all be considered as presentation dictates.

Specialist Opinions

There should be a low threshold for obtaining additional opinions from appropriate specialists:

--The consultation may assist with distinguishing the clinical importance of any symptoms or signs that may indicate underlying non-psychiatric illness that is beyond the assessing clinician's expertise.
--These opinions will help support a more confident diagnosis of a somatoform disorder if the specialist feels the symptom presentation is atypical.
--The patient perceives that a unified team of psychiatric and non-psychiatric experts is making the diagnosis.
--Involvement of specialists during the process of seeking a definitive diagnosis is more resource efficient in the long term than intermittent consultations for reassurance and infrequent but costly investigations.

Making the diagnosis

If after a very thorough assessment physical symptoms and signs remain unexplained, or are well out of proportion to any identified general medical condition, make the diagnosis of a Somatoform Disorder.
Use the following scheme to structure your thinking:

'Somatoform Disorder'
1. Physically manifesting as: ____________________
2. Probable cause/s of underlying emotional distress:
(a) Psychiatric syndrome: ____________________
As evidenced by: ____________________
(b) Psychological contributors: ____________________
As evidenced by: ____________________

This diagnostic schema and the rationale for its use is discussed in the previous chapter (pp. 29-31) and in more detail in Appendix I : On the Classification of Somatoform Disorders (pp. 154-6).

The full nature of the condition may not be apparent at the point of diagnosis, and aspects of the understanding of the underlying psychiatric and psychological components are often provisional. This is consistent with other complex psychiatric conditions in which the exact reason and timing for the clinical presentation is often not readily evident after initial assessment. The above schema will encourage the clinician to structure their understanding of the condition in a valid and clinically useful fashion, and it tolerates uncertainty and provisional diagnoses.

Preparing to share the diagnosis and transition to management of the condition

At the end of the assessment the clinician should treat, or arrange for optimal treatment of, any identified non-psychiatric conditions. When one or more colleagues are involved, the clinician should see to it that good communication occurs with the aim of optimal management.

What is the risk of diagnostic error?

Questions will and should arise about the likelihood of the risk of mistaking an atypical presentation of a non-psychiatric condition for a Somatoform Disorder. The clinician should be familiar with the historical and current rates of misdiagnosis in Somatoform Disorders. A review of the relevant literature is presented in Appendix II: The Risk of Misdiagnosis in Somatoform Disorders (pp. 161-3). After very comprehensive assessment, there remains a small risk of misdiagnosis, comparable to the risk of misdiagnosis in many common psychiatric and general medical conditions. This possibility of error should be shared with the patient, and, most important, should be weighed against the risk of *not* treating a potentially treatable disorder. All of these considerations are shared with the patient during the formulation.

References:

Waddell G, McCulloch J, Kummel E, Venner R: Nonorganic Physical Signs in Low-Back Pain; Spine 1980; 5:117-25

CHAPTER 5

FORMULATION

The Formulation

After your thorough assessment, draw together all of the data that you have gathered, and synthesize a clear understanding, in your own mind, of the patient's current predicament.

If a general medical condition explains all or most of the symptoms, the focus of management should obviously be on treatment of that condition. Your aim at this point is to share that information with the patient and the referral source, and to ensure that optimal medical care is facilitated.

If, however, the symptoms and signs are clearly *not* the result of underlying tissue pathology, or if symptom severity and degree of disability is clearly out of proportion to that which one would expect from the demonstrable tissue pathology, you are then in a position to make the diagnosis of a Somatoform Disorder.
If that is the case, notify the patient that you'd like to now have a meeting where you share the results of your assessment and discuss their future options. Schedule a time to meet.
At this meeting you will formally share with the patient your understanding of their condition.

Preparation prior to the formulation meeting

It is important to prepare well for this meeting, and to ensure that you have reviewed all pertinent history, clinical findings, and investigation results very thoroughly. Through this process you may discover that there is further information that needs to be sought out or clarified. Attend to that, if necessary.

No two patients with Somatoform Disorder are identical, and it is particularly important to customize the formulation to suit each patient. This customization takes into account multiple factors: the nature of the symptoms, chronicity, prior treatments, evidence for type of emotional distress, the patient's own attributions, degree of insight, and so forth.

Where possible plan to use the patient's own attribution theories and terminology

During your assessment, the patient's own theories of causation regarding the illness will have been specifically explored. An understanding of the patient's exact attributions are of critical importance when it comes to choosing concepts with which to share your own understanding of somatization in the formulation stage. Look for overlap in your conceptual framework of the illness and that of the patient's, and emphasize the commonalities. Attempt to meet the patient at that shared area of understanding, and to use that as a starting point to help them to begin to develop insight into the entire condition.

For example, elsewhere in the text (p. 101) there is a description of a patient who believed, with delusional intensity, that 'meridia' or 'energy lines' had 'tightened' in her body, decreasing her ability to move. In formulating an understanding of this patient's illness with her, it is wisest to initially look for overlap in the way that she conceptualizes the illness with our own best understanding of the pathophysiology. Rather than taking her to task regarding whether these 'meridia' exist or not, it is far more beneficial to work with her to integrate her concept of these structures with a basic understanding of Somatoform Disorder as brain-based illness with neurological connections to and from the periphery.

A similar approach may be used when patients have prominent beliefs about ways in which variables such as weather, diet, trivial injury, environmental 'toxins', and so forth may have caused or shaped their illness.

In a related fashion, while assessing the patient, you will have made note of the language that they use to describe their symptoms and physiological functions. If possible, use these terms, or variants thereof, in the formulation that you now share with the patient.

The formulation meeting

Adequate time, space, and quiet are necessary for this meeting. This may sound obvious, but it is an important consideration. Such clinical encounters can be watershed events in the treatment of these individuals, and clinicians should not attempt to supply formulations of this nature in an off-hand manner, or while rushed for time, or in inadequate space, for instance behind the curtains in a busy and noisy emergency room. Even though accurate, a formulation that is rushed is likely to be completely useless. So, approach the meeting with the gravity that it deserves.

The patient may elect to have people important to them present: family members, spouse, significant other or close support. Regardless of whether they initially choose this or not, it is wise to offer a follow up review meeting with the patient and their social supports, as we will discuss later.

If the assessment has occurred in a team or inpatient setting, it may be appropriate to have one or two other team members present. It is always important for the patient to be as comfortable as possible with the set-up at the meeting.

Validate the severity of the illness

Start the formulation meeting by reiterating your understanding of the severity of the illness, and how profoundly it has interfered with the patient's life. Discuss the length of time it has affected them, and show an understanding of activities that they previously enjoyed that the illness has now curtailed. Point out the differences in their pre-morbid and post-morbid levels of function.

Review your analysis of the symptoms and signs

Summarize the symptom and sign complex from which they are suffering, at length if necessary, integrating an understanding of the course of the illness into that review. This allows the patient to hear a review of their own story, and demonstrates again that you have considered and understood their experience.

Describe the logical steps that you have taken to exclude gross peripheral and demonstrable pathological causes of their symptoms. Review the different structures and systems that could be malfunctioning to cause such symptoms, and describe the ways in which you have excluded general medical causes for the symptoms.

For instance, in the case of a patient with a psychogenic paralysis of the right hand, review with them the ways in which muscle, joint, peripheral nerve, axillary plexus, cord/cervical spine, and intracranial gross pathology could all lead to such paralysis, but how you have managed to exclude those possibilities with physical examination and investigations (that in this case may include straight X rays, electromyography (EMG), nerve conduction studies, cervical cord imaging, and brain imaging).

In this analysis, also emphasize how results of prior assessments and prior investigations have been helpful in synthesizing the current understanding.

'The Brain is the Seat of the Illness'

Share the logical conclusion that the above analysis of their symptoms overwhelmingly indicates that the brain is the seat of the illness.

Discuss how your assessment has thus also included a careful search for possible structural pathology of the brain. List the commonly known structural brain pathologies that you have excluded with your assessment (physical examination and probable brain imaging), such as tumour, stroke, multiple sclerosis, etc.

If psychogenic seizure-like episodes are part of the presentation, at this point review the clinical, EEG and, perhaps, ambulatory EEG evidence for the episodes being non-epileptic in nature.

The illness involves brain function rather than brain structure

Share your conclusion that the illness is seated in the brain, and that rather than being caused by a clear structural pathology, it is caused by

an alteration in the way that the brain is functioning.
Reiterate that given all of the evidence, this really is the only logical conclusion that can be drawn.

Choose a metaphor or model as a way of understanding and talking about the brain illness

You have thus shared with the patient that the illness is based on brain function that has varied from the typical. At this point we usually introduce the use of any one of a number of related illustrative metaphors or models to describe to the patient what is likely happening in the brain to cause the illness. We suggest that you choose such a metaphor, and elaborate on it at this point. Some examples are discussed below.

The choice of metaphor is guided by the patient's own concepts regarding the illness, revealed to you during the assessment. In reviewing all of the data prior to the formulation meeting, you will likely have developed a good idea of the kinds of metaphors or models that may be most appropriate for this particular patient. This choice will also be shaped by the way in which the patient receives the understanding shared at formulation.

The metaphor or model thus chosen will serve as a way of talking about the illness through the management phase. Some of these models may sound mechanistic but they are all true to the principles of what we understand to be going on pathophysiologically in these conditions.
We do not yet have a full understanding of what exactly happens on a neurobiological level to cause and perpetuate a somatoform process, but we believe it is fair to conclude that (1) intact circuits are made to look dysfunctional when they are in actual fact structurally intact and capable of functioning normally, and (2) that areas or circuits in the brain that are not directly responsible for symptoms are likely dysfunctional as part or cause of this illness. Many of the models that we describe to patients make use of those ideas.

Examples of some useful metaphors and heuristic models

'Central', 'Brain based'
We commonly use these terms to remind the patient and reiterate that the brain is the seat of the illness.

'Running-interference'
"Your arm is paralyzed but the part of your brain that drives the muscles to your arm is intact, the nerves going to and coming from the arm are intact, the central switchboard receiving arm information is intact, all the important basic arm circuitry is intact. But there is something else 'running interference' with that circuitry, on a higher level of brain function, and that is the seat of the illness."

'Neurochemical changes', circuit 'dysregulation'
These terms may be useful for some patients, a hurdle for others. In some societies the stigma attached to psychiatric illness has propagated to a stigma against the sometimes euphemistically used '*chemical imbalance*'. Regardless of the exact semantics, one wants to relay to the patient that there is evidence for a change in brain function without an arguably more sinister change in structure.

'Hardware/Software'
Computer metaphors may appeal to some patients.

'Switchboard'
The brain acts as a 'switchboard' that both sends messages to the periphery and receives messages regarding how the periphery is functioning. 'Switchboard' malfunction can lead to the brain misinterpreting brain based illness as originating from the periphery.

Syndromes where dysfunction in one part of the body is misinterpreted by the brain to be originating in another part of the body.
Some patients may even allude to one or another of these syndromes during assessment or formulation, and they may find them particularly useful models for their Somatoform Disorder. Many other patients can benefit from learning of these examples of how the brain can deceive its owner regarding the origin of symptoms.
These kinds of syndromes include:
'Phantom limb': An amputated limb is still experienced to be present.
'Referred pain': Tissue pathology in one part of the body is experienced to be causing pain in another part of the body, usually because of shared peripheral innervation.
'Thalamic pain': A syndrome where a thalamic lesion causes a very severe peripheral pain syndrome, where no peripheral pathology actually exists.

Granted, some of these models may sound like overly simplistic metaphors, and they can also be criticized for possibly 'over-mechanizing' the patient's understanding of the condition. But note that each of them does indeed correspond with the broad way in which we understand the pathophysiology of these conditions. We continue to use them because they are effective: the vast majority of patients appear to find them to be useful cognitive frameworks around which to focus their treatment.

Metaphors may also prove to be useful in that they can reinforce to the patient how involuntary the process has been. The result of *'engine trouble'* rather than *'driver error'*.

'Vicious cycle' idea may be applicable

The idea that a *'vicious cycle'* is established in many forms of Somatoform Disorder, where central brain dysfunction sets up actual changes in periphery that then perpetuate the illness.

Increased muscle tone in a limb to brace against centrally originating limb dysfunction sets up muscles spasm and joint misuse that then cause peripheral source of pain. Postural change as the result of a somatoform illness may result in peripheral discomfort, then contralateral limb overuse, then musculoskeletal discomfort. Relentless focus and change in behaviours around physiological functions such as breathing, bowel movements, skin sensations, and many others, can have organic peripheral effects that then cause more symptoms and consequently perpetuate the syndrome.

Make it clear that the conclusions of the assessment means that a definitive diagnosis can be made

Many individuals with moderate or severe Somatoform Disorders will have been exhausted and demoralized by prior 'negative' investigations and (valid) opinions that there was no evidence of pathology in one or another of the body's systems. They will have had the experience of leaving doctors' appointments having been told that 'nothing is wrong' with one system or another. Point out that the current assessment has been comprehensive, and despite there being no evidence of significant causative tissue pathology on all tests to date, and *because* there is no evidence of such pathology, a definite diagnosis can now be made.

Give the condition a name

Share that all of the evidence leads you to conclude that they are suffering a condition know as a **'Somatoform Disorder'**. Explain that Somatoform Disorders are a group of conditions where 'brain-based distress is indirectly, involuntarily, and unconsciously expressed as physical symptoms'. For patients with developing insight, you may say 'brain-based emotional distress'. The patient will now have an accurate and valid diagnostic label for their condition.

You may want to add that the process by which Somatoform Disorders emerge is known as 'somatization', and that this process of 'involuntary physical expression of emotional distress' is common, complex, and involuntary.

It will likely be appropriate to also share that in different contexts, Somatoform Disorders may be variously labeled 'Conversion Disorder', 'Somatoform Pain', 'Somatic Symptom Disorders', 'Functional Disorders', or, even 'Hysteria'. It is usually important to proactively bring up these labels, as many patients will do their own research and come across writings linking somatoform conditions to various commonly used labels. It is better that they hear all of these terms from you in the formulation session, and bring questions they may have to you regarding clarifying their understanding of the diagnosis.

You may actively encourage some patients to do their own reading about their illness. At the same time, invite them to print out and bring any articles that they may want to discuss. There is much good information available on the internet but there is also a large amount of misleading information. Let the patient know this, and invite them to discuss any questions with you at future meetings.

If the patient suffers psychogenic seizure-like episodes, you may share that these can be described in various ways, including 'psychogenic', 'non-epileptic', 'pseudoseizures', or 'seizure-like episodes'.

You may share some literature with the patient about the condition. See our appendix 'Educational Information for Patients' (pp. 189-94) as a sample brochure that many patients find useful.

Allow for lack of complete 100% diagnostic certainty

Proactively point out that it would be naïve to assume absolute certainty in the diagnosis, but that, given the presentation and assessment process, and with the current state of medical knowledge, you are as close to certain about it as possible. We will often estimate figures like "90% certain", and we believe this is a fair estimate when current assessment techniques are used in a thorough manner.

One may want to emphasize that this is as good a degree of certainty, or better, as one gets in diagnosing many other medical conditions.

Reassure regarding ongoing monitoring

Reassure the patient that you and other clinicians involved in their care will continue to monitor their symptoms. If any features suggest a sinister change or emergence of underlying tissue pathology, you will investigate as necessary. Emphasize that at this current point there is no need for any further such investigation, and reiterate the diagnosis of Somatoform Disorder.

Validate the veracity of the illness

Emphasize that the illness is as real and as serious as any peripheral illness that may have incapacitated them in a similar fashion. It has, after all, disabled them as if it were such an illness. Again, point out the impact it has had on their lives.

Explain that the brain is the most complex organ in the human body, and that dysfunction of brain circuitry can present in very complex ways, such as the disorder they are experiencing.

Address any perceived delay in diagnosis

Somatoform conditions often present in complex and even puzzling ways, and it is not at all unusual for diagnosis to be delayed. Many patients will have gone through multiple assessments, investigations, and treatment trials for presumed illness, prior to eventually being diagnosed with a somatoform condition.

Acknowledge that it may have been frustrating for the individual to experience uncertainty regarding diagnosis for all this time, but that this is a consequence of the complexity of the illness. If the patient has gone through years of unexplained symptoms and medical contacts, this discussion point will be all that much more important.

Express unity with past clinicians, as appropriate

It is not unusual for patients with chronic somatoform conditions to displace some of their frustration with the illness onto prior caregivers. Address this directly. Point out that the current diagnostic conclusions have benefited from prior assessment, investigations and treatment trials. Point out that in many similiar situations you would have ordered similar tests and tried similar treatments. In many cases the prior assessments have served their purpose well, excluding sinister disease.

If a patient is particularly angry and blaming regarding past care, it is important to help them with this directly rather than ignoring these feelings. It is highly advisable to take care not to split with past caregivers. Apart from any such criticism likely being unfounded, splitting promotes blame and detracts from focus on management efforts. A patient's expression of anger and blame directed at others can also serve as another ego-defence; it may distract from focussing on more frightening underlying sadness or anxiety.

It is often useful to use the idea that 'the real villain is the illness'. This encourages the patient to move on and to direct their efforts towards managing the illness and improving their quality of life rather than lingering with blame and regret.

The condition is treatable

Point out that based on the diagnosis, you can tell them that they have a treatable condition. It may be appropriate to actively point out that the diagnosis is preferable to the general medical conditions that they previously may have feared or that may cause similar symptoms. Speak specifically about any such medical conditions if they have featured prominently in the patients concerns, pointing out that a somatoform diagnosis has a better prognosis in most cases.

Comment on underlying emotional distress

As noted in the 'Understanding' chapter (p. 31), the prognosis of the somatoform condition is closely related to the prognosis of the cause of the underlying distress. If at this point you believe there is strong evidence that leads you to be fairly certain of the form of the underlying emotional distress, you may be able to shape your discussion of prognosis with that in mind. Thus you may express varying optimism regarding prognosis depending on whether you believe the emotional distress to be related to, for instance, Major Depression, Psychosis, Personality Disorder, or transitory environmental distress.

Often, at this point, one is not yet sure as to the exact nature of the emotional distress, and it is always wise to keep an open mind in that regard. One's understanding of the form of this distress may change significantly over the course of treatment and ongoing longitudinal assessment.

Regardless of all these considerations, it is fair to emphasize that the condition is indeed treatable.

Remember that this may appear to be good news to you, the clinician, and indeed it is ultimately also good news for the patient, but a subgroup of patients with Somatoform Disorders will experience this news as threatening on some level.

> **Case Vignette:** *A 70-year-old woman had suffered incapacitating episodic psychogenic symptoms of various types, for more than 30 years. After thorough assessment, she was assessed to be suffering from a severe Somatoform Disorder. An understanding of her condition was shared with her while she lay in her hospital bed. At the point in the meeting where her clinician shared with her the news that this was a treatable condition, she immediately looked terrified and raised her knees up to her chest in a regressed and defensive posture.*

Thus, we must keep in mind that discussing potential resolution of the physical symptoms involves the suggestion that an ego-defence may be stripped away, and such news can be frightening.

Emphasize that the mechanisms are unconscious and involuntary, and that you know they are not malingering

Emphasize explicitly the unconscious and involuntary nature of the condition. By this time you will be able to state that you are aware that the patient is not causing the symptoms willfully. Emphasize that you know this to be the case. State explicitly that the condition is not a form of malingering.

The illness is not consciously caused, but the patient's efforts will benefit them in recovery

Work to frame the condition as an illness which the patient has not consciously caused or elaborated. While actively disavowing the possibility of the whole illness being driven by secondary gain, we also may point out any secondary reinforcers of illness behaviour. The patient is encouraged to see the benefits of recovery over any compensation or other factors perpetuating the illness.

Address the possible "Nothing is wrong/All in my head" concerns

When a somatoform formulation is shared with a patient, they may initially show some exasperation, as there are features of the understanding that may be a reminder of prior outcomes assessments. Patients may misinterpret the opinion to mean there is "nothing wrong", or that the illness is "all in my head".
These concerns should be explicitly addressed:
They have a definite illness.
A diagnosis is actively being made with this process.
The seat of the illness is indeed the brain.

> *"Yes, the illness is 'in your head' but only by virtue of the fact that your brain is 'in your head', not in the metaphorical sense of the phrase 'in your head': the illness is real and very definitely not imagined."*

Some patients are ready to entertain emotional distress as a causative factor at this point; others not

If the patient has already spontaneously volunteered that emotional factors may somehow be important, or if they volunteer that 'stress' may have contributed, or if they have used any kind of emotional language, you may be able to already start evoking 'emotional distress' as part of the mechanism. It may be useful to refer to the illness mechanism as a 'way in which the brain is expressing distress', or even a 'way in which the brain is expressing emotional distress'.

Again, validate prior suffering

When at all appropriate, validate the patient's prior suffering. We will often make encouraging comments regarding how they have bravely attempted to overcome the illness, but that the illness is so disabling that it has not been surprising that the patient's attempts have failed. We indicate this is evidence of the severe and involuntary nature of the illness rather than any lack of desire to recover on the patient's part.

Frame path to recovery; the patient has the ability to conquer the illness

Describe a potential path to recovery in such a way that the improvement is going to be a victory for the patient. The illness is serious but you believe they have the capacity to overcome it.

Use this as an opportunity to reiterate evidence of the patient's personal strengths that you have identified through the assessment process.

Reiterate that you will be supportive of them in their attempt to heal from the illness and improve their overall quality of life.

Meet again to answer questions and reiterate the major points of understanding

Give the patient time to 'metabolize' the information you have shared, and all of the implications. Second meetings for discussion of formulation are often required to ensure that any questions the patient has arising from all of those thoughts have been thoroughly addressed and discussed.

Being thorough in this regard *prior* to initiating any treatment ensures that a shared understanding is achieved. This shared understanding will be returned to, often repeatedly, during the management phase, and it is particularly useful to ensure that it is very clearly articulated beforehand.

Reiteration with spouse, family, caregivers, or other support present

Soon after formulating with the patient alone, it is almost always advisable to have a session where the major points of formulation are repeated for the patient, in the presence of their partner and other close family members.
This is clearly only done with the patient's consent, but is rarely omitted. One conducts the meeting as an advocate of the patient and with a view to facilitating sensible support from the family.
The understanding of the condition is laid out at such a meeting.
The involuntary and unconscious nature of the condition is emphasized. It is wise to explicitly state that the condition is *not* the equivalent of malingering.

The meeting is an opportunity to frame the illness in such a fashion that recovery will be a victory for the patient. Some patients overtly or covertly fear that recovery will prove them to have been previously deceitful; that if they recover, people will imagine that they were not 'really' ill. In many cases, they are aware of the great inconvenience that the illness has caused to those around them. It is important, in those instances, to emphasize that the illness is as 'real' as any involving demonstrable tissue pathology, and how the understanding achieved via the assessment now allows for a management plan that will allow healing. The clinician should emphasize any strengths the patient has demonstrated through the illness, and describe how those factors will help them work to recovery. Thus the clinician attempts to clear the path to recovery as thoroughly as possible.

Family insight into the overall condition is desirable, and leads to more appropriate support through the period of management and thus, a better prognosis. This is, however, often a complicated matter as family relationships have often been shaped by the illness, and in some cases, family stressors are part of the 'engine' driving psychological distress and the illness itself.

Allow the patient time to consider their options

After the formulation, give the patient time to digest the understanding you have shared. They will get an opportunity to clarify their understanding through questions and discussion at follow-up meetings.

Inform the patient that the diagnosis that has now been reached means that the illness is treatable. Certain treatments will have a good chance of succeeding in helping them overcome their illness.
Broadly sketch out the management you would suggest, customized to the specific patient's needs, based on principles laid out in the next chapter, 'Management' (pp. 83-125).

Suggested treatment may include regular out-patient visits (more rarely, inpatient care), medications, forms of psychotherapy, behavioural changes, and specific work with various medical professionals.
Give the patient the choice of proceeding. Allow them time to thoroughly consider their options.

Some patients will find the formulation unpalatable and decline the offered management. In that situation we recommend again ensuring that the patient understands the formulation. We would not want the patient rejecting the diagnosis out of misunderstanding. If the patient thereafter still declines treatment, we suggest 'leaving the door open'. Counsel the patient that they can contact you in future to meet again to discuss the condition, and that you would always keep an open mind about reassessing new symptoms. Emphasize that you would be available to help facilitate optimal care for them at a future date, if they should change their mind and wish to ask for treatment.
Write a comprehensive note describing the assessment, diagnosis and formulation to all medical professionals involved in the patient's ongoing care. State that you remain available to discuss the patient's situation and to see them again as needs be.
Some patients who initially decline recommended management will return at a later date and request care. It should be respected that some individuals require time to gain insight into their condition and to consider their options in light of the formulation.

Some patients prefer to try various alternative forms of treatment before trying those recommended by more orthodox practitioners. If patients improve with those pursuits, all well and good, if not they can return to discuss more conventional management with you thereafter.

If the patient decides to proceed with recommended treatment, one can then proceed to the management phase with the patient squarely in the 'driver's seat'.

Formulation Afterword:

The Formulation That Feels Overly Intrusive

In some situations it may feel intrusive to proceed with the formulation. This usually occurs when an individual suffering from a severe Somatoform Disorder has established a life around their illness that has the appearance of some stability and that, very superficially, may even seem fairly 'healthy'.

This adaptation to the illness may take many forms. From a physical perspective, the individual may have had their home environment very thoroughly adapted to accommodate their limitations. They may make use of special vehicles, hoists, elevators and various mobility aids. From a social perspective, family and friends may have made elaborate changes to their lives to incorporate the patient's illness. The patient may have also received special consideration from educational institutions or in the workplace. Some patients may even have become prominent public advocates for illnesses that they do not actually suffer.

In these situations, the physician may gain the strong impression that the act of sharing an understanding of the illness with the patient will be particularly intrusive, almost as though something will be 'broken' in the process. It is as though the careful balance that the patient has achieved with their illness in their life has something positive about it that is now at risk.

The idea that the illness is potentially treatable can itself be very threatening. Patients will often talk in terms of years of 'wasted' time, and may be anxious about the disruption of the current 'balance'.

> **Clinical Vignette:** *A 40-yr-old man, living in midwest of the United States, had a lifelong history of prominent dependent personality traits. While in an emotionally abusive relationship, he went through a period of increased psychological stress, and developed rapid-onset psychogenic blindness. By virtue of the blindness he received support from the community, gained a position working for an organization helping the disabled, and became a celebrated disabled artist. The clinical team who assessed him found themselves in a quandary about whether to proceed with formulation and whether to offer*

treatment. They feared that the diagnosis and treatment would possibly be more detrimental to the patient than simply letting him continue living as he had been with the existing disability.

It is our opinion that the assessing clinician and team are obliged to proceed with the formulation. We believe that is the right thing to do, no matter how elaborate or superficially 'healthy' the adaptation may seem.

There are a number of reasons to do so:

1. Moral and professional obligation to share your honest and truthful opinion with your patient.
2. Even though it may not be initially obvious, the individual is suffering very significantly at some level. After all, they are seeing you for assessment. Thus, their apparent adaptation may only be superficially 'stable'.
3. An argument can also be made that you are legally obliged to proceed.

Whenever we have found ourselves in this position, we have reason to pause and consider what is best for the particular patient - but we have in all cases then proceeded to formulate an honest understanding with the patient.

CHAPTER 6

MANAGEMENT

The Management of Somatoform Disorders

The focus of the treatment of Somatoform Disorders is to help the individual suffering the condition to achieve resolution of their physical psychogenic symptoms, while at the same time treating their underlying emotional distress and any other manifestations of psychiatric illness. It is important to continually keep in mind the two major components of the condition. Throughout, one continues to help the patient to improve their insight with regard to the process of somatization.

Customizing treatment to each patient is of central importance. We have attempted here to share many facets of our approach, in the hope that you can choose to incorporate techniques that suit a specific patient's needs as well as your own therapeutic style. In this chapter we will elaborate upon psychological, pharmacological and physical treatments that we have found to be effective. We will also share specific strategies and broad principles useful in helping individuals with Somatoform Disorders. You will simultaneously be considering and using the following modalities of treatment:

Psychological and behavioural interventions (p. 85)
Pharmacological and other biological interventions (p. 96)
Physical therapies targeting psychogenic symptoms and conditioning (p. 106)

all the while keeping in mind

Broad principles (p. 110) and
Specific situations (p. 121)

During the assessment and formulation phase, your understanding of the nature of the patient's underlying emotional distress will have developed, and your initial treatment efforts will be determined by how you view their dysphoria. Does the patient suffer a major endogenous psychiatric condition such as Major Depression, Panic Disorder, or Generalized Anxiety Disorder, in which symptom patterns and neurovegetative changes signal significant dysregulation of brain circuitry? Or is the patient experiencing a more reactive type of emotional distress, where an interaction of personality, coping style, and current life circumstances is resulting in dysphoria? Or is there a combination of causes?

Proceed to help the individual with similar techniques to those which you would utilize in other patients with similar causes of emotional distress. Aim to use the same treatment techniques you would use if the core emotional distress was more overt and the main presenting concern. Consider the type of psychotherapy and pharmacotherapy, used independently or in combination, that you believe may be most beneficial given the nature of the distress.

If the distress appears to be more the result of psychological processes, make more use of psychotherapeutic techniques.
If the patient has clear evidence of psychopathology related to an endogenous psychiatric disorder, with associated neurovegetative changes, medications are likely indicated.

Even if there is evidence that an endogenous disorder is the main engine driving the psychogenic symptoms, ongoing educational, supportive, cognitive and behavioural psychotherapeutic techniques will most likely be vital in assisting the patient with complete recovery. Medications alone seldom resolve all symptoms.

Pharmacotherapy can sometimes help the patient make use of psychotherapeutic techniques. Judicious use of medications targeting, for instance, sleep disturbance, excessive anxiety, or depressive symptoms may result in improved capacity to initiate behavioural change or engage in psychotherapy.

Develop a stepwise, flexible plan

You may choose to initially emphasize a psychotherapeutic approach, and suggest an introduction of medications if either neurovegetative symptoms become prominent or empirically if, after weeks or months of psychological treatments, there is little progress. Or you may decide to attempt a trial of medications early, targeting any neurovegetative features. It is not uncommon for one's understanding of the source of the dysphoria to evolve further during treatment, and treatment strategies would then change to incorporate that changing understanding.

At the same time as using pharmacological and/or psychological therapies for the underlying distress, use physical therapies to treat the manifest physical symptoms and for overall reconditioning and rehabilitation.

Ultimately, the aim of management is to improve the individual's overall quality of life. With a sensible, tenacious, stepwise approach, the majority of individuals will experience a reduction or eradication of psychogenic symptoms, improved psychological functioning, and consequent improved quality of life.

Psychological and Behavioural Interventions

Psychological work is customized to patient and clinician factors

All clinicians have personal preferences regarding the types of psychotherapeutic approaches that they find most useful. Use techniques that make sense to you, and that you have found to be helpful for other patients with similar forms of emotional distress.

One can use combinations of educational, supportive, behavioural, and cognitive techniques. Take into account the patient's attribution theories, world view, education, intellect, and degree of insight. Behavioural interventions regarding daily structure, exercise and sleep are often very helpful.

A psychodynamic understanding of the patient will inform aspects of the way in which one directs therapies, but a purely psychodynamic approach to treatment is not recommended, particularly early in the therapy. Patients with somatoform conditions tend to respond better to active supportive, cognitive, and behavioural techniques. The very act of interpreting the physical symptoms as being psychogenic is in itself challenging to their somatization ego-defence, and is thus anxiety provoking. The patient will likely require support around dealing with that. We recommend avoiding other ego-defence challenging psychodynamic interventions, particularly early in the therapy.

Continue to emphasize the understanding of the condition

During the management process we reiterate aspects of the formulation very often. One wants the patient to have a clear understanding of the nature of the somatoform process such that they can begin to see that the physical symptoms are indeed treatable and can consider the possibility of covert emotional distress driving their condition. Thus a good portion of ongoing treatment consists of educating the individual thoroughly about their illness.

For some patients, the concept of 'stress' affecting the brain is helpful. In others a mechanistic discussion of neurotransmitters and dysregulated circuits effecting motor or sensory circuits may make most sense. In hyperkinetic functional movement disorders and non-epileptic seizures, patients may benefit from the model of an averse and excessive reaction to a specific emotional state or threat. Review the various models discussed in the section on formulation (pp. 69-71), and consider which may best suit your patient.

The cognitive framework for understanding the condition, presented in the formulation, and shaped over time with the patient such that it makes sense to both the patient and the treating clinician, is the core model to which you return during the months (and sometimes years) of treatment. Effectively, this is the core cognitive therapy of the condition. This change in core belief also facilitates use of treatments that will actually address the condition, and the subsequent improvement in function and quality of life.

Sample therapist statement:

> "We know that your symptoms are very definitely the result of brain function.. there's no other possible explanation for the symptoms... and at the same time we know that they fortunately aren't the result of any sinister or obvious brain pathology, such as a stroke, or a brain tumor... the pattern of the symptoms, the scans, and the other investigations show us that. And that's all good news, because there is every reason to believe that your illness is treatable... there is no evidence that you shouldn't be able

to overcome these symptoms entirely. I know they've been present for years, and that this may sound like a stretch in view of that, but there really is a very good chance that they can settle completely."

Sample therapist statement:

"Now, as we've discussed before, what is happening is that emotional distress is being expressed in an indirect fashion.. through these physical symptoms... The circuits that are responsible for [limb movement/co-ordination/normal limb functioning] are all completely intact. But emotions are 'running interference' with those circuits, and, when we get that interference to stop, the limb will be freed up to function completely normally again."

Sample therapist statement:

"As you know, these episodes you're having are not epileptic seizures.. they aren't the result of abnormal electrical activity in the brain. We know that because the EEG shows that there is no epileptic activity during an episode. The 'pseudoseizures' or 'psychogenic seizures' that you're having (we could choose to call them either), are the result of emotional distress emerging in this indirect fashion. You also have panic attacks, and in fact, the psychogenic episodes are probably best thought of as another form of panic attack, or another example of a pathologic and excessive reactivity of the nervous system. They're another way in which the emotional distress is making itself known.

Sometimes it's useful to think of this using the metaphor of the toothpaste tube: you have a build-up of emotional distress, like toothpaste building up pressure in a toothpaste tube, the cap is on, and you aren't sure how to safely name or talk about this feeling of stress, or what to do about the stress, so the toothpaste finds another way out. It squeezes out through a hole in the bottom of the tube. That is what is happening if you have a pseudoseizure. The stress emerges in the form of a pseudoseizure. Instead of the pressure expressing itself as a panic attack, or instead of you being able to tell yourself or your wife: "I'm anxious; I'm feeling very uncomfortable; I'm feeling stressed". Instead of that, the stress emerges as the seizure-like episode. That's why we also call it a 'conversion disorder'; the emotional stress is 'converted' into physical symptoms.

So, a central task in healing from this illness, is for you to learn to keep the cap off the toothpaste tube. You need to learn to identify that feeling of distress, so that when it surfaces, when the pressure builds, you are able to say to yourself: "Hey, I'm feeling anxious". You can share that realization with your wife, and you can tell me about it, too. You can lay it out on the table, and face the fact of the matter, that at times you feel anxious and stressed. And that's fine, that's an important step. It may feel scary at first, but there are many ways in which you can learn to decrease the emotional stress. And, in this way the seizures will stop entirely. There'll be no reason for the toothpaste to squeeze out the back of the tube."

Ongoing Longitudinal Assessment

The understanding of the patient and their condition may well change over time; be prepared for that. The initial assessment, even though it will have been comprehensive, may turn out to have been a 'reconnaissance flight', and new information may change the way the patient understands the underlying emotional dysphoria, the mechanism for the symptoms, or other aspects of the condition. It is often not until the patient fully recognizes the likelihood that their symptoms are psychogenic that the antecedents of the condition can be properly appreciated.

Clinical Vignette: *A 63-year-old school teacher had suffered from a chronic pain condition precipitated by a soft tissue injury in a motor vehicle accident 30 years prior. In the first year of treatment she endured significant grief recollecting how she had misattributed the pain to the motor vehicle accident and her body's failed ability to heal, rather than to important emotional factors in her life at the time. She then made progressive gains in her physical and emotional functioning after she appreciated how the accident had changed her approach to coping with certain emotional states and induced a state of behavioural inhibition within her relationships with others.*

Be prepared to accept that one's initial impression about the underlying cause of the patient's emotional distress may have been inaccurate. Emotional distress that was initially thought to be the result of a major affective disorder may be determined to be psychologically rooted, or vice versa. The meanings of certain symptoms may become apparent as one learns more about the patient's past, and their personality and world view. The importance of cultural context may become apparent.

Further history may emerge, as the patient's trust is gained. In some situations, information about substance use and abuse are revealed and shed light on the presentation. Certain symptoms may have been held back by the patient in the initial assessment, out of guardedness or embarrassment or lack of trust; symptoms regarding obsessions, or grooming disorders, or eating disorders, or sexuality, for instance. There are also times when overt delusions may only become apparent during longitudinal assessment.

Any such new information will be useful in understanding the patient and their condition that much better. Continue to explore the emotional states that may have precipitated the original and ongoing symptoms. Encourage the patient's attempts to better understand those antecedents, and explain that they may not have seemed to be important at the time their physical symptoms first developed.

Clinical Vignette: *A 23-year-old medical student developed persistent post-concussive symptoms after a minor head injury. She had difficulty reconciling how she may have developed somatoform symptoms when her life appeared to be improving for the better at the time of her injury. After several weeks of reflection, she recognized that she had started a new relationship just prior to her injury, after a period of relative avoidance of intimacy due to a previous difficult break-up. She had again become markedly avoidant of intimacy after her injury and attributed this to her head pain and other difficult physical symptoms. When she addressed her challenges with relationships through psychotherapy, her physical and emotional symptoms improved.*

Keeping the 'basket' of symptoms together

It is very common at the end of the assessment to have a list of symptoms affecting various systems and various parts of the body that are all judged to be psychogenic. It is important during the formulation process to ensure that each of these symptoms is clearly discussed with the patient and that the management that then proceeds includes this entire 'basket' of symptoms. If only one or two central symptoms become the focus of the treatment, it is not unusual, months later, to find that other symptoms have been 'left behind' as they have not been conceptualized as part of the entire syndrome by the patient. Sometimes such symptoms will spontaneously resolve along with recovery in the core emotional state and the most obvious physical symptoms; at other times, however, this will not occur spontaneously, and the patient will be left with residual symptoms. Thus, the recommendation is to frequently reiterate all symptoms that are targets of treatment.

Emphasize that the central physical symptom is not the only target of treatment

Patients may be aware that the broad extent of their disability goes well beyond that attributable to their most obvious physical symptom. They may consciously or unconsciously fear that somehow therapy would be terminated if one or two central physical symptoms settle. The clinician should be aware of this possibility and in some cases be very explicit about educating the patient in this regard: should certain central symptoms resolve completely, therapy would continue in view of the broader and still disabling condition. In a related vein, the patient may fear that once their physical symptom resolves they would be considered completely well. Discussion of the importance of both physical and non-physical symptoms (those affecting emotions and neurobehavioural function) emphasizes to the patient that one is targeting overall recovery, and that they would not necessarily be expected to be fully functional if their physical symptoms resolved rapidly.

Enhancing patient motivation as a major factor in determining positive outcome

In the treatment of many psychiatric disorders, good patient motivation is closely associated with positive outcome, and this is also the case in recovery from Somatoform Disorders. Factors particular to these conditions, however, may hinder a patient's motivation.

The nature of the condition may be challenging to understand, and as a result it may be unclear to the patient how and where to apply their efforts. Thus, the importance of ongoing education and use of a clear cognitive framework in the ongoing therapy.

Assisting the patient in increasing their motivation to regain health is often a delicate matter. We do believe the somatization process is primarily an ego defence and therefore, on some level, the individual is to be expected to unconsciously resist the resolution of their physical symptoms. Their ability to reduce the need for this unconscious defence is going to depend on a reduction in the underlying emotional distress as well as a cognitive framework that allows them to alter their beliefs regarding the physical symptoms.

Many sufferers will have gone through periods where they felt somehow blamed for their condition. There is also the danger that the patient themself may assume that if a condition is emotionally based they are somehow at fault for its development. And when it comes to assigning blame, some patients will reveal persistent anger directed at agents that they believe have caused or worsened their predicament: circumstances of injury, insurance companies, or past medical caregivers. This is where active psychotherapy will be very useful, to help the patient deal with guilt and anger, and to redirect their energies to be more completely focused on healing. Again, the 'villain is the illness' idea can be useful to the patient.

Patient motivation and responsibility

We believe that we are most helpful to our patients as almost unconditional advocates, and will support them to great extent in their endeavours within the different domains where they are trying to make their way: the health care system, their families, and various educational, occupational and social contexts. We would hope for and expect the same from our own medical professionals should we find ourselves in a similar predicament.

Yet at the same time, we are aware of the fact that the patient's own personal internal motivation will correlate very highly with a positive outcome. So we want to support the patient while at the same time assisting them in developing independent strength. This is a delicate balance. On the one hand, too much support and advocacy may encourage inactivity and dependence, and hinder progress; on the other hand too little support will likely not assist the individual in their recovery, and may even recreate the neglect and abandonment that individuals may have experienced by being misunderstood in their illness.

As an ego-defence, somatization is argued to be a relatively 'immature' way of dissipating emotional distress. Furthermore, people tend to regress in illness, even more so when that illness is chronic and treatment resistant. So the 'load' that a patient with significant somatization may be capable of bearing may initially be very limited.

There is what may superficially appear to be an internal paradox to the message we give to a patient suffering a Somatoform Disorder: the onset has been unconscious and involuntary, but the emergence from the illness will be assisted by their own motivation and conscious efforts. This may initially appear internally inconsistent, but is not. The difference is that, with the formulation shared by the clinician, the patient has the opportunity to understand their condition in a new light, and it becomes clearer to them how particular efforts can gain traction.

We will often use the idea of "80% effort" in the various domains of rehabilitation. The idea here is that the patient should extend themselves to a point where they are carrying a reasonable load, but they should not overextend themselves. Indeed, some patients, at assessment will be found to have been overextending themselves very severely in misdirected attempts to force themselves to 'get better' - overly strict or onerous regimens of routine, exercise, diet, or cognitive endeavours. Thus, the guide through recovery is to use "80%" effort and not "110% or 120%".

The challenge is to help the patient to carry almost the heaviest load they can at each point in their recovery, but not too much. Too much and they will be overwhelmed, and will likely pause or regress.

A very welcome and important change that can come about in treatment is for the patient to gain a sense of agency, with increasing sense of control of their circumstances. This will not result from them being told that they have agency, but rather from them seeing that that are capable of activities and tasks that they had previously not been able to execute. They will benefit from having their clinician point out these improvements, and appropriately label them as the patient's victories. The therapeutic benefits of small incremental improvements in actions should never be underestimated. This is why attention to basic behavioural techniques can be so useful in assisting recovery: daily routine, weekly schedule, sleep routines, regular sensible nutrition, and a modest number of scheduled activities.

Target complete resolution of physical symptoms

In situations where absolutely no medical cause has been found for physical symptoms that also have psychogenic qualities, it is fair, even in chronic illness, to have as a treatment target the complete recovery from the physical symptoms. This may seem overly ambitious, but it is a position that results from the experience of having seen individuals with very severe chronic symptoms recover from those symptoms. It can thus be argued that with every patient the clinician should consider an initial trial of tenacious therapy aimed at as complete a recovery as possible.

We thus strongly recommend one avoids counselling one's patient that you'll help them "learn to live with their disability". Such a conclusion may lead to premature closure and consequent treatment nihilism in patients that could potentially have improved.

After very thorough trials of therapies, usually over more than a year or more of management, a small percentage of individuals may prove to be truly 'treatment resistant', but this is not a label that should be applied lightly as it may lead to the cessation of potentially helpful lines of treatment.

Chronicity of symptoms is often seen as a barrier to complete recovery. This may be a genuine concern in that disuse of a limb or long term avoidance of physical activity may, rarely, have had permanent effects on a patient's musculoskeletal function. But even in chronic illness the goal should remain to restore the patient to maximum health as the underlying psychiatric condition is in most cases treatable.

Prepare the patient for changes in physical symptoms

If any new physical symptoms emerge, assess them with an open mind, in the same thorough way the presenting symptoms were approached. Sometimes one will work with a general practitioner or a specialist physician to assess new symptoms thoroughly. State openly in your recommendations to your colleagues that any new physical symptoms should be assessed as in any other patient (somatizing patients tend to engender a more nihilistic approach to medical care in practitioners).

Depending on the nature of the therapy, developing transference may now make it less appropriate for the treating therapist to repeat physical examinations that were done in the initial assessment.

Advise patients that physical symptoms may be temporarily exacerbated when one is taking a more active approach in their treatment. Reassure the patient that new physical symptoms will be assessed as necessary.

Introduce the idea that 'nobody gets better in a straight line', meaning that occasional set-backs are to be expected in any recovery and should not be seen as 'returning to square one'.

Ensure that the patient knows that alleviation of physical symptoms is a central goal and that an important part of that is the alleviation of underlying emotional distress. Patients may lose motivation when they do not see their physical symptoms readily improving despite positive changes in their mental and emotional state and functioning. Reassure them that the nervous system often takes time and practice before manifestations of aberrant functioning appear to change.

Encourage the patient's development of insight

Patients differ greatly in their degree of insight at initial assessment. Some may be in complete denial about the possibility of any form of emotional distress contributing to their illness; others may, at the very first meeting, volunteer thoughts about the effects of "stress" or "anxiety" contributing to their physical symptoms.

Some patients arrive at a psychiatric assessment ready to hear that their physical symptoms are the result of emotional distress, but even after thorough assessment, mental health clinicians may be reluctant to confidently make the diagnosis of a Somatoform Disorder. A lack of very obvious overt psychiatric or psychological causes may understandably act as a major deterent to drawing the logical conclusions. Sometimes the nature of the underlying distress only becomes apparent during therapy, once the somatoform defence has attenuated and emotions emerge.

Clinical Vignette: *A 48-year-old woman with a three year history of a psychogenic movement disorder underwent a thorough* *neuropsychiatric assessment. She received the formulation hesitantly. After a two-week hiatus, she returned to the clinic with a very thorough understanding of the psychosocial stressors that had culminated in her inability to manage anxiety and cause her physical dysfunction and sleep disturbance. This enabled her to be highly motivated in her recovery and her insight continued to develop independent of professional intervention.*

Through successful management, the patient comes to understand how emotional distress plays a central causative role in their illness. Share a psychological understanding of the somatoform defence with the patient when the time is right for that individual. For some patients, insight may only develop over months or even years of treatment.

Emergence of more obvious psychiatric syndromes

As somatic defences fall away and physical symptoms improve, do not be surprised to see the emergence of more obvious psychiatric syndromes. Treat these as you would similar symptoms in any other patient. Assist the patient in understanding what may for them be frighteningly overt emotional distress. Explain it in terms of the overall model. One does not want to encourage catharsis for its own sake, as there is no evidence that that is beneficial. However, when more direct emotions emerge as the somatic symptoms settle, it is persuasive information and this formulation (of the 'de-conversion', if you like) should be shared with the patient.

Clinical Vignette: *A 42-year-old married woman had suffered from involuntary movements for several years. After multidisciplinary inpatient treatment had begun settling her physical symptoms, she began to disclose that she was engaging in new and increasing repetitive and deliberate self-harm behaviour including sexually acting out. Her emerging behaviours were addressed as a novel attempt to contain emotions that were distressing and unfamiliar to her.*

Couple and family involvement

It is often useful to have at least occasional meetings with the patient's partner (if they are in a relationship) and other family members. At these sessions educational points can be reiterated and progress can be described. If progress has been slow or as of yet is non-existent, this can be framed in the context of the complexity of the disorder.

Specific couple or family work may at times be helpful, particularly in situations where it is determined that psychological distress and interpersonal functioning is an important part of the engine driving the somatoform condition. Sometimes a few sessions with you, the patient's primary clinician, may be helpful. In situations where you determine that more thorough couple or family therapy is necessary, it may be important to have an independent therapist offer that care in parallel with your ongoing work. Here again clinician preferences and skills affect decisions.

Even if direct psychological work with the couple or family is not indicated, the patient and their support system will likely benefit from hearing your thoughts about how their patterns of relating to each other have effected the shape of the condition, and your ideas about how their support can assist the patient's recovery.

Pharmacotherapy and Other Biological Interventions

Use of medications in Somatoform Disorders

Special attention needs to be given to considering the rationale for use of medications in the treatment of Somatoform Disorders.

In mild forms of Somatoform Disorders, one may be able to avoid the use of medications altogether, and patients may achieve resolution of symptoms with psychotherapeutic interventions alone. In moderate to more severe forms of the condition, medications are very frequently indicated. We only consider use of medications when careful analysis leads us to believe that the potential benefit of a medication significantly outweighs the risks of a trial of that same medication.

It can be a difficult decision, whether or not to make the suggestion to embark upon use of medications. In our opinion, the most useful point regarding this judgment, is whether we ourselves would want to use medications if we were suffering the same disorder. Thus, with all we know of the patient's condition, of these disorders in general, and of the efficacy and side-effects of available medications, would we want to take medication in this situation? Many clinicians use such a threshold in guiding their recommendations, and it is a sensible approach. Share this thinking openly with the patient.

Sample therapist statement:

> "I understand why you don't take this decision lightly; neither would I. But, if I were suffering the same illness that you have, with everything that I know about these illnesses and about the treatments, I would at this point attempt a careful trial of a medication."

Understanding the reluctance towards use of medications

Some patients suffering from a Somatoform Disorder may be willing to accept the idea of at least some 'stress' or 'emotional distress' as being part of the illness. That subgroup will usually more readily accept the idea of using psychotropic medications aimed at assisting the underlying emotional distress aspect of the disorder.

In another group of patients, however, the somatoform process is so complete that it hides all insight into the presence of emotional distress or prominent psychiatric illness. That, after all, is closely related to the primary unconscious purpose of the somatization defence - to alleviate experience of the underlying dysphoria. These patients will, naturally, be less likely to see the need for psychotropic medications. They will understandably see no rationale for using medications for symptoms that they don't consciously experience, or see to be primarily important.

Thorough education around the nature of the condition is an important part of introducing the idea of using medications. You may already have shared the idea of certain aspects of brain function 'interfering' with intact circuitry. If there are related neurovegetative changes, those symptoms can be used as evidence for dysregulation of basic brain circuitry. If an individual has problems with any combination of energy levels, sleep, appetite, libido, weight change, motivation, and speed of thought or movement, it can be put to them that changes in these basic human functions ("animal level" functions, as we'll sometimes say) are evidence of basic neurobiological change, and that it is fair to consider medications that may assist those circuits and, in turn, those functions.

Even after such an explanation, it is still very difficult for many patients to entertain the use of medications. Many have educated themselves about the realistic challenges of using medications; just as many will have misconceptions about the risks. Many will have imbued medications with all sorts of sinister and even magical qualities, instead of seeing them for what they are: potentially useful tools. Many misconceptions may be related to the patient's attribution theories and their understanding or misunderstanding of body physiology. There is no substitute here for very thorough education: regarding the medications themselves, the indications for their use, the target symptoms, the various medication options, the effects and side effects of each. This is time consuming work, but, in the long run is worth every minute. Ideally, informing and educating the patient very thoroughly will allow them to be able to assess the effects of medication trials as objectively as possible.

Clinicians who work to help patients who have high anxiety levels are well aware of the acute sensitivity that many have regarding the side effects of medications. A subgroup of patients with Somatoform Disorders are anxious and hypervigilant regarding any physical symptoms. They are highly prone to misinterpret physical symptoms at the time of medication use. Symptoms of the illness can be misattributed to medication side-effects. It is important to introduce medications very gradually in this group, and to see the patient relatively frequently to assist them with placing any change in physical symptoms in proper perspective. In some circumstances, the patient's effort to avoid any physical distress from medications represents a similar mechanism to the emotional avoidance subserved by the somatoform defence, and this may be a potentially fruitful avenue of exploration into the utility and consequences of avoidance behaviour.

Over and above all of these considerations, the stigma regarding use of 'psychiatric' medications pertains to those with Somatoform Disorders as much as any other group of individuals suffering psychiatric illness. This should be addressed directly when it arises. Fortunately there has been significant progress in many societies over the last 40 years regarding an increasing acceptance that psychiatric disorders are as real as any other medical condition. It is, nonetheless, still very important to acknowledge to patients that ignorance regarding psychiatric conditions remains widespread, and to emphasize how clear it is that these illnesses are indeed real, and that they are rooted in disturbances of function in the most complex organ in the body, namely the brain. Comparing use of psychotropic medication in brain-based illnesses to general medical examples, such as antihypertensives for idiopathic hypertension, and insulin for diabetes, can be useful.

Use of medications is determined by features suggesting a neurobiological pathophysiology to the underlying emotional distress

If underlying emotional distress appears to be predominantly psychological, the product of who the individual is, and how they find themselves responding to their current life circumstances, we will emphasize using psychological and psychotherapeutic interventions more prominently than medications. In that context there still may be place for limited use of medications to attempt to treat depressive symptoms, excessive anxiety, or sleep disruption.

If there is definite evidence of a syndrome such as a mood disorder, an anxiety disorder, overt psychosis or any other major psychiatric diagnosis, and where there is prominent insomnia, we will introduce the idea of using medications more readily.

In almost all individuals with definite insomnia we will use behavioural techniques around sleep hygiene, and daily exercise, in conjunction with simple hypnotics to attempt to improve sleep pattern. Written daily and weekly schedules, though seemingly simple, are often very useful.

Any prominent evidence of markedly increased baseline anxiety or panic attacks we will most usually treat with introduction of a serotonergic agent, sometimes in conjunction with benzodiazepines. For definite Major Depression our usual stepwise approach is similar to commonly used guidelines. For any individual with a strong family history of Bipolar Affective Disorder or a personal history suggestive of any prior episodes of hypomania or mania, we will more likely make early use of mood stabilizers.

Note that all of these approaches are in keeping with how a clinician would approach treating psychiatric syndromes where the emotional distress is overt. Your medication choices are based on what you assess to be the core cause of emotional distress.

A stepwise, symptom-driven approach to the use of medications

Medication choice is based on knowledge of which agent is most likely to benefit the symptoms that are most impeding the patient's emotional function and quality of life. Matching an agent to the most intrusive symptoms is preferable to attempting to categorize the symptoms, and then using a standard treatment for such a category. It is far better to keep in mind each of the symptoms that one is treating, and to make use of a medication best suited to that symptom constellation.

Thus it is better to focus on, for instance, the individual symptoms of depressed mood, insomnia and daytime lethargy, than to summarize those symptoms as 'Major Depression' and treating as if for that broader category.

One will have in mind a stepwise plan, as in "if agent 'x' is not helpful, I will add agent 'y', and then, if there is no response, change to a trial of agent 'z'." Share with the patient that this is your approach, and that you are making medication choices based on current knowledge of which agents are likely to best help their exact constellation of symptoms. Share with the patient that the science of these choices is imprecise, and that there consequently may be some trial-and-error to the process. Emphasize that ineffective medication trials are not necessarily indicative of misdiagnosis.

The initiation of a stepwise medication trial is the beginning of a journey to find a good fit between the patient and a medication regimen that works. Sometimes, by good fortune, a person may respond rapidly. At other times, it may take tenacity and many steps to find a good fit. It is good to prepare a patient for either eventuality.

Use of dopamine blockers in patients with somatoform disorders

Good support for anti psychotics

The use of dopamine blocking agents in patients with Somatoform Disorder deserves separate and specific consideration, as it can be controversial to use an antipsychotic agent in the absence of very definite positive psychotic symptomatology. This deserves specific mention as their use for these conditions may be interpreted to be 'off-label' in some countries.

There are two valid arguments for using these agents in a subgroup of individuals with Somatoform Disorders. The first is the theoretical argument that many individuals with Somatoform Disorders can technically be considered psychotic in that they have a strong somatic beliefs that have all the features of delusions - they are 'fixed false beliefs'. For instance, an individual may believe their arm is paralyzed when in fact it is not paralyzed. Some would argue that by virtue of this conviction the individual can be considered psychotic and it would thus be fair to consider use of a dopamine blocker in their treatment.

The second major reason for arguing for use of these agents in some patients with somatoform disorders is largely based on clinical anecdotes. The authors and their colleagues have worked with patients where we have ardently attempted psychological and pharmacological treatments, short of dopamine blockers, for periods of 6, 12 or 18 months who have then responded rapidly over 6 to 8 weeks to the introduction of low dose dopamine blockers. There does seem to be a subgroup of patients who benefit from these agents and, indeed, may actually require dopamine blockers in order to resolve their somatoform symptoms.

All this being said, most clinicians in our group choose to use dopamine blocking agents only later in treatment, and only if other regimens have failed.

In a less challenging fashion, there are some individuals who from the time of the initial assessment, by virtue of the nature of their symptoms, can be clearly seen to suffer a psychotic disorder. It is then fair practice to recommend use of dopamine blockers early in the treatment.

> **Clinical Vignette:** *A 30-year-old nurse had a roommate who developed tuberculosis such that she herself was required to take triple prophylactic therapy. She developed a persecutory psychosis almost definitely secondary to one of those agents, that led to her believing that 'meridia' or 'energy lines' in her body inhibited her behaviour in a number of bizarre ways. These included the inability to stand still for even a moment (despite being able to walk, sit and lie down) as well as a belief that if she elevated her hands above shoulder level, 'meridia' on the left side of her body would pull on her heart in a dangerous fashion. These beliefs were completely fixed and*

were judged by her assessing clinicians at the time of assessment to be symptoms of a psychotic disorder. The individual was bedridden and was disabled to the point that she needed to be helped with feeding. Her illness and all of the physical symptoms resolved within 2 months of commencing treatment that included risperidone.

The use of narcoanalysis for diagnosis and treatment

In some circumstances, almost always in an inpatient setting, narcoanalysis using sodium amobarbital (amytal) or midazolam may be highly advantageous for both diagnostic and therapeutic purposes.

This procedure is best suited to individuals with symptoms that impede motor function. For instance, it is well suited to individuals with paralysis of one or more limbs, an unusual psychogenic gait disturbance, psychogenic speech abnormalities, and in some instances psychogenic movement disorders. It is not well suited to symptoms that are not visible or negative symptoms, for instance, pain syndromes, or visual or hearing deficits. Techniques inducing disinhibited states are of only limited use in certain forms of Somatoform Disorders, for instance, those creating unwanted movements such as tremors. Such symptoms will almost definitely decrease or even resolve with use of sedating agents, but the meaning of such a response will be far less profound than the restoration of function where none previously existed. In episodic somatoform conditions, such as in an individual with non-epileptic seizures, there is usually no place for these techniques.

The principles of the treatment are to disinhibit the individual in such a way that the cognitive framework necessary for the maintenance of the psychogenic symptoms is 'released' and previously paralyzed or otherwise disturbed motor function normalizes. The procedure is also well suited if the individual has very limited insight into the nature of the condition, as it can be used to inform the individual in a dramatic fashion of the reversible nature of their condition.

Narcoanalysis is performed in a controlled environment in a unit that is attached to a general hospital and is equipped with services required for resuscitation should there be any medical difficulties during the procedure. Over more than 20 years of using this procedure and many dozens of applications, we have on no occasion had to use emergency resuscitation. Amytal or midazolam is administered intravenously with the patient sitting or lying comfortably as appropriate for the physical disability. Present in the room we will have the treating clinician, the patient's most trusted nurse, professionals involved in physical rehabilitation such as the occupational therapist or physiotherapist, and on occasion, family members. The patient gives informed consent for the procedure and informed consent to have a video camera running throughout the procedure to record any progress they may make. For some individuals we will also administer a stimulant such as methylphenidate 10 mg 30 to 60 minutes prior to the sedative to attenuate any unwanted somnolence that the amytal or midazolam may cause.

The idea of using narcoanalysis should be introduced to the individual in a very direct manner with the stated purpose of revealing that this is the same substance that in the past has been nicknamed "truth serum" and used in interview techniques attempting to elicit hidden information. Emphasize that the procedure is not being used in an attempt to somehow reveal anything that is consciously hidden but rather to inhibit the process that is in itself running interference with the normal circuits serving the patient's periphery. Thus, formulate the use of amytal as something that will transiently remove that interference. Again this metaphor is broadly consistent with the way in which we see this procedure to be functioning. Draw up 500 mg of sodium amytal or 10 mg of midazolam and administer it at a rate of sodium amytal 50 mg/minute or midazolam 0.5 mg/minute. If this is administered too slowly one does not get the disinhibited response and if administered too quickly it may actually make the individual too somnolent.

Once the patient is under the influence of the sedative as evidenced by mild somnolence and most often the onset of nystagmus or mild dysarthria, briefly interview them with regard to how they are feeling. Disinhibition is sometimes evidenced by laughing or giggling.

The main part of the procedure is focused on the afflicted body part. In the case of a paralyzed limb work with the individual to attempt to get some movement of the limb. For the sake of the video, which they will be asked to watch carefully the day after the procedure, examine them before and after administration, getting them, for example, to lift and move the limb attempting to get some evidence of increased muscle use with the sedative. Any such increased movement will be recorded on the video and can then be played back to the patient afterwards, often with profound effect. If an individual has a gait disturbance, get them to walk with assistance while disinhibited; if they have speech disturbance, get them to repeat spoken phrases, and so forth.

Thus the major idea of the procedure is to attempt to get even a small amount of function of previously dysfunctional body parts such that the patient can view this progress later. Narcoanalysis, used in this fashion serves as a form of immediate cognitive therapy, as it can immediately replace the longstanding belief "I am ill" or "I am injured" with the belief "I am suffering but my condition is reversible." In addition to having diagnostic and treatment effects as described, suggest to the patient that activities during narcoanalysis allow their intact brain circuitry to begin to practice functioning normally again. Note that during the procedure interference is removed or partly alleviated, and this allows the circuit that has been inhibited for so long to commence action again. This cognitive framework is a useful step in the recovery process for many individuals.

As an alternative to narcoanalysis, consider use of modern video cameras with 'night cam' settings to record video (with the patient's informed consent) of them while they sleep at night. This video footage produces a similar effect to conscious sedation in that limbs that are held paralyzed through waking hours are seen to be moving during sleep and thus it can be revealed to the patient that basic motor and sensory circuitry is intact to the limb, and this, in a similar fashion to use of narcoanalysis, can allow the patient to commence recovery. Seeing is, for many patients, believing. Others who have accepted the diagnosis by the weight of the formulation and the evidence behind it, without any demonstration of the reversibility of their deficit, may still benefit from the physical work facilitated during the disinhibition of narcoanalysis.

One should be aware that for a small subgroup of individuals, the process of watching a video of a previously dysfunctional limb working during narcoanalysis can be an emotionally traumatic experience. In effect the process strips away an ego defense in a very dramatic fashion. Be sure to be particularly supportive of the patient through this process and aware of the possibility of emotional regression or deterioration as a consequence. For a small subgroup this can be the reverse of the "conversion" process, with the primary gain of somatization being reversed and them experiencing psychic distress as a consequence.

Clinical Vignette: *A 68-year-old man with a thirteen year history of pain and dystonia following a mild muscle strain while walking into work, received 8 mg. of midazolam during narcoanalysis. He reported to the video camera that his pain was substantially attenuated and his range of motion in his neck and affected shoulder improved considerably. Upon reviewing his video with the nursing staff, he indicated that he did not believe what he had said as he was "under the influence of drugs", and that his range of motion improvement was probably coincidental (describing periods in the past when he had experienced brief remissions). His lack of trust for the treating team and his entrenched belief that he had been injured were refractory to pharmacological treatments and 3 months of intensive cognitive therapy. He remained disabled by a conversion disorder with an apparent associated delusional disorder.*

Optimize medications previously instituted for presumed somatic indications

At the time of being diagnosed with a Somatoform Disorder, many patients will continue to be using medications started in the past, when their physical symptoms were thought to have general medical causes. These medications may include antiemetics, bowel motility agents, muscle relaxants, analgesics, anti-vertigo agents, anti-allergy agents, and many others.

When a thorough assessment has shown that the patient's symptoms are likely due to a somatoform process, we recommend slow weaning from these medications. Reduce agents slowly and in a stepwise manner, prioritizing the withdrawal of agents that are more likely to have detrimental side effects first. Emphasize that it was fair to have had trials of these agents at the time, given the symptom complex, but that the assessment at this point suggests that such medications are unlikely to be useful or are only partly useful in treating the underlying illness. We often specifically state that if we had been the patient's treating clinician in the past, we may well have attempted trials of similar medications. We do this because some patients will be distracted from the task at hand with regrets about prior trials, and we would emphasize, in the vast majority of situations, that those trials were worthwhile steps in attempting to treat their complex condition.

All biological therapies are used in the context of ongoing psychological work

While a decision may be taken to attempt a stepwise trial of psychotropic medications, it is at the same time important to continue use of psychotherapeutic techniques. Ongoing support and education are essential, and amongst other benefits, will almost definitely improve medication compliance. Ongoing psychodynamically-informed cognitive interventions are likely even more beneficial. Ultimately, all interventions aim at decreased emotional distress, behavioural change and improved quality of life.

Physical Therapies

Using physical rehabilitation techniques and specific physical therapies can be particularly helpful in treating many patients with somatoform symptoms.

Targeting general 'reconditioning' and activity schedule

Any individual suffering a subacute or chronic condition becomes inactive and 'out of shape' as a consequence of the condition. Inactivity causes loss of muscle strength and bulk, decreased flexibility and range of motion, as well as decreased cardiopulmonary fitness. In Somatoform Disorders, this 'deconditioning' may be particularly obvious, and out of proportion to underlying physical potential. Inactivity will in many cases have been driven by a conviction that physical symptoms make exercise impossible or intolerable. The avoidance of physical activity can at times be part of the patient's overall strategy of avoidance and hence physical therapy may also be a form of psychotherapy in that it encourages gradual exposure to an exaggerated or misperceived threat (often the threat of worsening a perceived physical condition).

In any patient where activity levels allow, we recommend encouraging them to commence a gentle stretching and exercise regime, steadily building up in frequency, duration, and intensity. Often we'll recommend this informally, and monitor progress at follow up sessions, but at times may recommend that a patient see an appropriate professional to help them with such a program.

This work can potentially be done by a physiotherapist, an occupational therapist, a rehabilitation physician, an activity specialist, or any one of a number of other 'hands-on' therapists focusing on improving physical function. Personal trainers or fitness instructors may also be able to play a pivotal role.

Guidance regarding healthy nutrition, and where appropriate, focus on weight reduction may also be part of such a regimen.

Many patients benefit from the introduction of a weekly activity framework, where planned activities including exercise and recreation are mapped out. This may be particularly beneficial to patients who have been unwell for long enough to have lost all weekly routine. It is also helpful for those who have experienced loss of regular sleep patterns.

Like all behavioural changes, an increase in physical activity may exacerbate somatoform symptoms particularly if they are perceived as putting the patient at increased risk of a potential threat (e.g. once I get more active, I may need to return to work, or interact with specific individuals, etc.). Patients should be advised of this typical response in advance and be supported through it if it occurs.

Physical therapies targeting specific psychogenic symptoms

Physiotherapy, or various other forms of direct physical therapies, are used to specifically focus on somatoform symptoms: parts of the body where the patient may be experiencing weakness, reduced range of motion, loss of co-ordination, hyperkinetic movements, or pain.
Focus of that care is recovery of physical function, and it can be critical to successful outcome.

It is important for the professionals applying the specific physical therapies to be aware of the psychological underpinnings of the patient's disability. It is most helpful if these members of the treating team have experience working with Somatoform Disorders. If that is not the case, then you, as the primary treating clinician, should try to spend time with those individuals sharing very thoroughly your understanding of the nature of the patient's condition. It is important that the physiotherapist is aware that Somatoform Disorders involve symptoms that are inconsistent with typical patterns of pathophysiology, and that they are not put off by that fact. It is very important that the illness is understood as being real, and that the process of symptom production is seen as unconscious and involuntary.

There is a risk that professionals without experience with these disorders may approach them as though they represent a form of malingering, and patients very rapidly become aware of that fact and respond poorly. Thus, close communication between you (the treating clinician) and any professionals involved in physical therapies is paramount. It is important that all professionals helping the patient are using the same basic model regarding the nature of the condition and the expectations regarding management and recovery.

There is a good chance of a useful synergy occurring between the psychological therapy and the physical therapy. In the psychological work, the treating clinician emphasizes how the peripheral physical systems are intact and potentially able to function normally; and how the brain circuitry responsible for function of those systems is intact. In the physical work, these ideas are built upon and tested repeatedly. During assisted range of motion work or in gentle exercises, the therapist will point out evidence of normal or improving function. For instance, any evidence of muscle strength in a previously weak limb is a physical example of the intact 'circuit' beginning to function normally again. This is evidence to the patient and the therapists that somehow the interference is settling, and that normal function is recovering. The treating clinician should also monitor this in brief serial examinations during regular sessions.

The physical therapy may become a form of psychological behavioural therapy (gradual exposure or behavioural activation with the recognition that this does not worsen but rather improve the condition) and cognitive therapy (the understanding that the condition is not primarily physically based). Active as opposed to passive therapies are recommended so the patient can develop greater sense of self-efficacy.

Breakthroughs in treatment often come in a session of physical therapy. It is important that the physical therapist is aware that pacing should be largely determined by the patient and not the therapist. Often patients will regress if they feel pushed too fast or too hard in behavioural and physical therapies.

Clinical Vignette: *A 19-year-old woman with psychogenic quadriplegia that had required total care for six months, was admitted to an inpatient neuropsychiatric ward for assessment by a multidisciplinary team. She was seen by a neuropsychiatrist, a physiotherapist, a social work counsellor, a neuropsychologist, an occupational therapist, and numerous skilled psychiatric nurses. The therapy that followed included psychotherapy, psychotropic medications targeting underlying anxiety and depressed mood, as well as various physical therapies. The therapeutic breakthroughs came in physiotherapy sessions, where hands on physical therapy and assistance demonstrated to her that her limb function was returning and she was able to commence what turned out to be a complete recovery.*

Even though not the primary intention, the emotional effects of 'hands-on' therapies such as physiotherapy and massage can play a role in 'mobilizing' the physical and the psychological factors inhibiting physical function. We don't specifically aim for such effects, but we are aware that they may be active.

While physical therapies are being actively used, it is wise, in the psychological therapy sessions, to mentally prepare the individual for possible substantial breakthroughs. In particular, the patient must learn that it would not be seen as odd for them to suddenly improve, as this happens in the treatment of Somatoform Disorder treatment fairly often. People are most familiar with disease patterns that require substantial time for recovery. A person who has a hemiplegia from a stroke doesn't suddenly get better in their third physio session. But individuals with Somatoform Disorders can make such breakthroughs, and shouldn't be held back by beliefs to the contrary. So it is wise to prepare patients and their families for possible sudden improvement.

Sample therapist statement:

"I know it's challenging to do some of these exercises at present, but give them a try each day. Don't push yourself too far... 80% effort is a good limit to use. If one exercise feels like too much effort, try

the others. And do the same with walking... try to walk each day as planned, but don't overdo it. Even if you do overdo it a bit on some days, you won't injure yourself irreparably with the exercises."

Sample therapist statement:

"There are many ways in which people improve. Nobody gets better in a straight line; there are often small setbacks, that's to be expected. Often there will be an hour or a day or even a week where it feels like you've taken a step back. Don't get demoralized by that."

Sample therapist statement:

"It's impossible to predict exactly what your path to recovery will look like... some people get better at a steady pace, others may get sudden breakthroughs. So, for instance, you may suddenly notice that the range of motion of your elbow suddenly increases in one of your physiotherapy sessions. Don't be alarmed by that, many people get better with that kind of sudden step. Remember that the circuits controlling the muscles in the arm are completely intact, and once interference settles, your arm will be freed up to work normally again. Sometimes that happens suddenly."

Broad Principles

Through the treatment process, follow these broad principles:

Therapeutic alliance

An effective working alliance between the individual suffering from a somatoform condition and their treating clinician is central to successful outcome. It is important that the patient knows that the treating clinician sees their condition as real, and that they trust them to be open, honest and supportive.

Quality of therapeutic alliance, along with the patient's motivation to engage in using offered treatments, are possibly the strongest prognostic factors for successful treatment.

Tenacity and ongoing care

Successful treatment often requires persistence over months, or even years. This is particularly true for individuals who have chronic symptoms. It may take numerous steps in a therapy before any kind of improvement is noticed in emotional, neurovegetative, or physical function. It is important to be tenacious in one's approach to treatment, as some individuals do well after initial periods of apparent treatment resistance. Thus, be prepared for ongoing care. Neither you nor the patient should be too disappointed by periods of plateau, or minor setbacks; they are to be expected.

Reinforce gains

Positively reinforce improvement. Frame gains in the patient's functioning as a victory for the individual, and use the fact of the gains to further nurture the patient's motivation to improve further. Educate the patient and significant family supports regarding these gains in a supportive fashion. When appropriate, emphasize the fact that the observed gains support the diagnostic formulation.

Be an advocate for the patient

It appears to be helpful if the treating clinician also acts as a sensible advocate of the patient, within their family, social and occupational domains. This may involve the completion of required paperwork describing the condition for institutions such as schools, the workplace, insurance companies, and others.

Allow the patient to lead the way

It is particularly helpful if you, the treating clinician, are able to allow the patient to have a sense of control over their management direction and the 'speed' of treatment. It is for this reason that it is important that the patient begin treatment willingly and without any sense of coercion. Emphasize that they are "in the driver's seat" regarding management decisions, and that you will offer guidance and recommendations. Attempts to force individuals to adopt management plans that make no sense to them almost always results in poor outcome.

Return to work issues

Allow the patient space and time with regard to return to their occupation; this approach is usually more efficient in the longer term, and will almost always result in the patient returning to full function sooner than if they had been pressured to attempt to do so. Here, again, allowing the patient to lead the way usually results in better outcome. The approach to return to work goes to the heart of the clinician's understanding of the process of somatization. It challenges one's beliefs regarding the unconsciousness of the process, the patient's motivation, and the concept of secondary gain. It is important that all members of any defined management team co-ordinate well regarding work expectations. It is our opinion that if a patient is an active participant in their own recovery, then they should be an active participant in their decision to return to work. It is advisable to openly discuss the benefits and risks of a return to work, and any tendency to avoid the work environment. Complicated situations arise when a patient is not actively seeking therapies yet expects excusal from work. One should not mandate therapies (especially if they have been tried and have not proved useful). If third parties do mandate treatment we find that this is rarely useful. At the same time, the reality of external return to work expectations can be helpful in motivating some patients.

Managing anger & frustration

It is common for patients, early in the assessment or initially in the management phase, to express exasperation, frustration and even anger at the apparent lack of a definitive diagnosis and recommendations in the past. It is important to recognize this frustration as there may have been many situations during which the diagnosis was in fact unclear or ambiguous, or the patient felt blamed for their condition, or in which honest and well-meaning but futile efforts were made to alleviate their suffering. Often, patients experiencing grief and anger will elicit frustration in the care provider and may be labelled as difficult. As the current treating clinician, you may be targeted as part of the service/health providing team that is perceived as inadequate. Validate the many difficult setbacks and ambiguities that have complicated a thorough understanding of the condition. Blame the condition itself for its complexity and avoid attributions of criticism to those who merely did their best to help the person function. Help the patient understand that the way in which they responded and the misattributions they made were understandable given what was known about the condition at the time. Refer to how the nervous system initially misled the patient and clinicians alike into believing the problem was disease-based or peripheral rather than functional or central. Redirect the patient's grief and anger in a useful direction in terms of the possibility of future recovery.

Anger directed at past caregivers

It is important to recognize early the patient who is highly critical of prior medical caregivers. There is a risk of interpersonal splitting if the assessing clinician does not deal with this in an active fashion (see p. 74).

Express the opinion that the prior assessments and investigations were appropriate and necessary at that time, and the data from them (even 'negative' or inconclusive results) are useful now. Indicate that the thorough review of the records has allowed one to do this.

It is often useful to point out that many of the medical steps taken in the past were necessary at the time, even though they seem in retrospect to have not been immediately productive. We will often explicitly state that had we assessed them at that earlier time, we may well have come to the same conclusions, or ordered the same investigations, as were done in the past.

Through these methods of framing past medical experiences, one can usually redirect the patient's energies to the task at hand, namely understanding and managing the illness.

Importance of good intra-team communication

Communication within the outpatient or inpatient team should be optimized. A consistent approach is essential. With outpatients, keep in good communication with all treatment providers to ensure the broad principles of management are adhered to. With inpatients, regular meetings amongst the sometimes extensive management team are essential. Inevitably there are times when communication is suboptimal as it is almost impossible for all members of the treatment team to be informed of all recent developments at all times. Effective discussion of complex cases helps to improve providers' attitudes, as it is common to encounter feelings of helplessness or therapeutic nihilism in the more challenging clinical situations.

As in many situations in the treatment of severe emotional health disturbances, complex somatoform illness can apply complex psychological challenges to the cohesion of the treating team:

> **Clinical Vignette:** *A 43-year-old labourer with a twelve year history of disabling fatigue asked for the nursing staff to remove the lid from his lunch tray as he felt the consequence of doing that himself would be prolonged pain and fatigue for the rest of the afternoon. In an attempt to encourage his recovery, the treating nurse asked him repeatedly to try to do this on his own and expressed disbelief to the treating team that he was unable to complete this task, especially given other inconsistencies in his physical abilities. Other nursing staff agreed that this felt demeaning to them. A team meeting was necessary to discuss what would be reasonable expectations of the patient given that he was digesting the formulation and had been encouraged to consider at what pace he would start to expose himself to tasks that provoked his symptoms.*

The issue of clinician motivation and ambivalence

In attempting to help individuals with moderate or severe Somatoform Disorders, there will commonly be circumstances during the management phase when some or all of the members of the treating team question whether any progress is being made. This usually stems from the complexity of the condition.

Ambivalence within individual treating clinicians is also common. This often turns on whether there is a factitious or malingering component to the patient's presentation, or whether the patient is showing significant motivational challenges. Through the assessment, the clinician assesses the patient's relationship with their syndrome, and their specific symptoms. The differentiation between a somatoform and malingering/factitious disorder is based on the clinician's judgement. If the clinician believes that the patient believes they are ill in this way, then the disorder is somatoform. There are no special tests to differentiate; it is a matter of clinical judgment. Revisit this understanding if ambivalence is encountered. Ask the team or onself: "do I believe that the patient believes that they are unwell?" If answered in the affirmative, this should focus thinking, and encourage the clinician and treating team to persist in moving forward and helping the individual with their recovery.

If there is clear evidence of a factitious illness, this should be addressed in a direct and open manner with the patient. Obviously this is not a diagnosis to be taken lightly, and is usually made on the basis of very clear evidence. The clinician should lay out the evidence for conscious elaboration of symptoms, as well as any obvious deceit. Offer to organize psychotherapeutic help for the patient if requested. Such formulations often end at that point, with the patient abandoning the assessment and any offered management. Share your diagnostic impression with the referral source, the family practitioner, and any other medical professionals who have been involved in care.

Addressing prognostic factors in the management phase

The course of a somatoform condition usually follows the course of the underlying causative psychiatric or psychological condition, rather than anything particular about the exact physical symptom presentation. Thus, very severe physical symptoms such as psychogenic blindness or psychogenic quadriplegia may have a good prognosis if they are the result of underlying emotional distress that is amenable to treatment. Conversely, an apparently relatively minor physical symptom, such as the reduced range of movement of a limb, may have a very poor prognosis if it is related to underlying emotional distress that is chronic and treatment resistant.

A percentage of Somatoform Disorders may turn out to be completely treatment resistant but in our experience, this represents a small minority. The majority of patients, even those with severe conditions, will experience at least partial remission of physical symptoms and assistance with underlying emotional distress if they make use of the management suggested above. What is particularly important to note is that tenacious management can produce complete resolution of physical symptoms and good control of emotional symptoms in many situations that may initially have appeared intractable (to both the clinician and the patient!). Ideally, all patients for whom somatoform symptoms are impeding their quality of life should be offered this management approach.

Chronicity itself can make illness more intractable. Habits of illness behaviour can become entrenched and make management that much more challenging. Even though chronicity often results in an initial hopelessness in the patient it should not lead to therapeutic nihilism for the clinician.

Somatoform Disorders can persist for long periods if the underlying dysphoria is chronic, or if physical symptoms persist out of habit even after the underlying emotional 'engine' spontaneously settles. In each of these situations thorough assessment, formulation and a systematic stepwise approach to management can achieve surprisingly good outcomes. It is thus important to keep an open mind even in seemingly unfavourable situations. This is especially the case in situations where there have not been prior trials of psychotherapy or pharmacotherapy aimed at somatoform illness.

Stepping in with a straightforward formulation and sensible use of psychotherapy and medications can sometimes have very rapid positive effects. It is important in these situations to prepare the patient and those around them for the possibility of rapid gains.

The 'Virtual' Outpatient Multidisciplinary Treating Team

Patients with Somatoform Disorders would likely best be treated by formal multi-disciplinary outpatient treatment teams. This would allow for tight communication within the team, and ideal co-ordination of management efforts, which would result in optimal treatment. Unfortunately, such arrangements are rare, and in most parts of the world funding limitations and lack of political will have restrained their development. We would hope that an increased awareness of the prevalence and impact of Somatoform Disorders would motivate participants to develop such clinics in the future.

As it is at present, clinicians are left to develop multi-disciplinary teams spread out across the community, customized for each patient: 'virtual' teams, if you will. In our own system, such a team usually consists of the treating psychiatrist/neuropsychiatrist, the family doctor, a physical therapist (most commonly a physiotherapist), an activity specialist (most commonly an occupational therapist), as well as any other practitioners that the patient may require because of their specific needs. Some patients will also receive treatment from psychologists, counsellors, and mental health teams.

In this kind of arrangement, the treating clinician becomes the 'switchboard' or 'quarterback' in co-ordinating the team's management direction, and this requires considerable effort and time spent with written, telephone or other communications.

An alternative method is for the clinician to forego attempts to co-ordinate a 'virtual team', and to rather accept the system as a 'black-box'. In this scenario, the clinician puts all of their efforts into their sessions with the patient, makes recommendations regarding other forms of therapy that may be helpful, but also accepts that the patient will be continuing to have diverse contacts with the medical system and other caregivers over which the clinician has little influence. The hope is that any other therapies pursued by the patient may contribute to improvement, and if not, that as the patient improves they will see less need for pursuing treatments that are not addressing the core causes of their illness. The disadvantage of this approach is that other health care providers may be offering models of understanding the illness that are at odds with the one offered by our clinician, and this will likely hamper progress. The advantage is that if this approach ends up resulting in effective treatment, it is far less labour intensive for the individual clinician (but not necessarily more efficient from a system-wide perspective). If this approach is assumed, it is suggested that an explanation is provided to the patient that any therapies that reinforce that the underlying cause for the disorder is physical and not emotional should be used with caution as they may slow recovery and worsen prognosis. The patient's attempts to continue to seek care that focuses on physical diagnoses is understandable and one would want to empathize with that desire while continuing to share with the patient the understanding of the illness that has resulted from your assessment.

Setting for Management

Treatment can take place in either an inpatient or an outpatient setting. The exact context within which management is offered will be determined by the severity and chronicity of the condition, the nature of one's clinical practice, and the accessibility of the patient to the treatments offered, including geographical distance. For less severely impaired individuals with access to a clinic, outpatient management is recommended.

The vast majority of patients can be treated on an outpatient basis. It is advisable to set up a series of frequent outpatient appointments, the more frequent the better: initial weekly appointments would not be excessive.

Treatment on an inpatient ward is suggested for those who are very severely functionally compromised, and as a result require daily medical and nursing care, and frequent physical therapy. Inpatient care also allows the treating clinician to meet with the patient on a daily basis during the commencement of treatment. This can greatly expedite initial treatment steps. Formulation can be reiterated as necessary, questions answered, and, if medications are being used, any emergent side effects can be quickly addressed.

It can be particularly challenging to set up adequate care for individuals who live at a distance. It usually takes a large amount of effort on the part of the assessing clinician to share a comprehensive and nuanced understanding of the individual with clinicians in the periphery in order for treatment to proceed successfully. Such a plan also requires that clinicians in the periphery are familiar with using this model of treating these disorders. Although resource intensive, a period of hospitalization can make a critical difference in the recovery of an out-of-town individual who is suffering with a moderate to severe Somatoform Disorder.

Addressing the use of 'alternative' therapies

In many parts of the world various therapies labelled 'alternative' may be readily available, and a good number of patients will independently decide to pursue such treatments. This pursuit is often a reflection of the fact that they have found their symptoms unresponsive to initial orthodox treatments through primary medical care. Our broad approach is to embrace any techniques that offer persistent improvement. "Whatever works" is a fair mantra. At the same time, we are honest with patients about our opinions regarding these therapies, and also emphasize that we are unable to unreservedly endorse them; many do have risks.

Some alternative therapies do appear to demonstrate positive treatment effects for some patients. Most evidence suggests that these positive effects are the result of non-specific elements (a caring therapeutic alliance, plus placebo effect). These therapies may also be indirectly useful by encouraging functional activation or by offering a convincing narrative that allows the patient to step away from physical symptoms.

Reinforcing the holistic approach

So much lip service is paid to the grand concept of 'Holistic Care' that the term has almost become a meaningless piety. That said, there really is no way of effectively helping individuals with Somatoform Disorders without being genuinely 'holistic'. The clinician should be very broad and comprehensive in both assessment and management. Biological and psychological factors are of equal importance, as we have repeatedly emphasized. In addition, a nuanced understanding of the patient's values and world view, including cultural and religious perspectives, will be invaluable when it comes to assisting them with their symptoms. It is important to thoroughly understand the patient's beliefs about their condition, in order to be able to frame the treatment in a manner that makes sense to the patient.

Treatments that focus solely on the patients' biological functioning, such as pharmacotherapy without consideration of psychological or social contributing factors, and that fail to thoroughly understand the meaning of the condition to the patient, are unlikely to succeed.

> **Clinical Vignette:** *A 58-year-old woman had endured over twenty years of stimulus sensitivity, chronic fatigue, and multiple chemical sensitivities. Involuntary eye closure associated with acute light sensitivity had resulted in functional blindness. Years of psychoeducation and supportive therapy, in addition to courses of antidepressants and antipsychotics had provided benefit but without any associated functional gains. She was admitted for a course of ECT which led to a further partial improvement. Once behavioural therapy and marital therapy were introduced, it became clear that previous therapeutic efforts had most likely contributed to, not helped her confront her pervasive avoidant tendencies, and she subsequently made progressive gains in terms of her symptom burden and her functioning.*

> **Clinical Vignette:** *A 50-year-old mechanical engineer suffered debilitating illness since his twenties. Symptoms were multitudinous,*

and included atypical abdominal pain (for which he had received numerous surgeries and procedures), atypical chest pain, unusual peripheral pain syndromes, chronic headache, very severe insomnia, and, more recently, non-epileptic seizure-like episodes. He had been completely disabled for 5 years prior to admission, and was using opiates at the equivalent of 1000mg of morphine per day when he was admitted to a neuropsychiatry unit for assessment. Very thorough history taking, examination, and investigations revealed lifelong deep dysphoria and no definite evidence of peripheral cause for his pain. Couple and family assessment in parallel with the above revealed that his wife was a very caring medical professional who had been a very strong advocate for her husband, and his family life had been completely governed by his health needs. In one family meeting his son volunteered: "I've only known my father through his illness", and recounted memories of driving his pain racked father to ERs in the early hours of the morning. Once the findings were formulated with the family, they went through a period of being less supportive, but couple work and family work continued nonetheless. Evidence for underlying Major Depression became obvious, and the patient was weaned off all opiates and treated with antidepressants and dopamine blockers. Depression and insomnia initially persisted but then responded well to a course of ECT. All symptoms improved greatly with ongoing use of medications and physical exercise in the form of longer and longer walks. Non-epileptiform seizure-like episodes abated. Family became more supportive again, but less closely so than during the worst of the illness. It became clear that, along with lifelong dysphoria and recurrent Major Depression, the patient also had significant dependent character traits. His condition stabilized on pharmacotherapy, psychotherapy, and basic reconditioning with him returning to good active daily routines but never able to return to work. Twenty years later he remains pain free but is starting, at the age of 70, to run into challenges with degenerative osteoarthritis.

Interclinician variability in aspects of treatment

Using this model, a treating clinician will do their very best to understand the nature of the emotional distress underlying the somatoform condition, and will then attempt to assist the patient in alleviating that distress. All clinicians are aware of the inter-clinician variability that exists within psychiatry. This is a challenge for our field but also a reality. Despite the fact that we all learn partly-standardized methods of assessing patients, there remains a good deal of inter-clinician disagreement when it comes to attempting to assess, for instance, whether an individual is suffering a mild biological depression or a psychological demoralization in response to life circumstances. Any clinicians reading this who work in teams and get opportunities to discuss diagnoses with their colleagues will be acutely aware of this. Thus, identical patients may initially be offered different specific treatments depending on the clinician that they see. Some clinicians will be more likely than others to see biological underpinnings to a symptom of dysphoria, other clinicians more likely to see the psychological causes of the same distress. If all clinicians entertain both hypotheses, and use stepwise approaches, patients will ultimately respond well regardless of the clinician's initial specific approach. All clinicians using this model, will be aiming at alleviating the patient's underlying dysphoria, reducing the physical symptoms, and, ideally, helping the patient develop an understanding of the process of somatization.

Specific Situations and Techniques:

Treating Somatoform Pain

Pain is a highly personal experience, and is modified by individual and cultural variables. It is a very challenging symptom to address.

A thorough assessment and search for general medical causes is essential in all patients with pain as a presenting feature. One must be thorough in attempting to understand whether the pain is caused by tissue pathology, or whether it follows the pattern of any known neurological pain syndromes. That said, pain is one of the most common somatoform symptoms and in most such circumstances occurs in the presence of other somatoform symptoms, therefore giving further clues to its etiology.

In the course of the treatment of a somatoform condition, the recommendation of therapeutic behavioural activation and desensitization in someone experiencing significant pain is often met with disbelief and may appear to be paradoxical. Yet increased activity is often the key to improvement.

Cognitive behavioural therapy with guided relaxation, activity schedules, sleep hygiene, and cognitive strategies for dealing with pain flares and analgesic use, can all be helpful. Serotonergic agents, tricyclics, and dopamine blockers may be required. Physiotherapy can assist with local changes secondary to pain, such as increased muscle tone.

If a somatoform pain diagnosis is made, patients using prescription opioids will be encouraged to undergo a cautious and purposeful weaning off these medications if at all possible. We are aware that this may feel like a tall order, and even paradoxical, in individuals who have been using morphine, codeine, demerol, fentanyl, hydromorphone or methadone for long periods. However we do believe that each of those agents is not useful in treating the root causes of somatoform pain and believe there is good evidence that they may actually worsen syndromes such as depression, anxiety and insomnia. Opioids also psychologically reinforce the belief that the condition is physically based, and mask otherwise highly treatable psychiatric symptoms such as panic attacks. Analgesia that reinforces a state of avoidance also contributes to the patient's passive state, implying that only a medication, and not anything they can do, will modulate their nervous system. Thus, although it may feel like a daunting task, we recommend weaning from these agents. In extreme cases this may require inpatient admission. A myriad of clinical examples illustrate the effectiveness of this intervention.

Clinical Vignette: *A 45-year-old teacher was referred by her gastroenterologist for assessment of very throughly investigated atypical abdominal pain that did not appear to be due to any abdominal pathology. Over 5 years of this illness she had been using ever increasing doses of opiates, initially codeine, and then morphine. Her history was compatible with a Somatoform Disorder, with moderate to severe recurrent Major Depression driving her dysphoria and, most likely, her abdominal pain. With psychotherapy, antidepressants, and the dopamine-blocker olanzapine, she was able to wean off the opiates and greatly improve her overall function. Her pain decreased to the point that she would have periods of weeks and months pain free. Over 15 years of follow up she relapsed and sought use of opiates briefly on two occasions but her overall function remained better than prior to the somatoform diagnosis. Despite steadily increasing insight, she remained at ongoing risk of using opiates to "throw a blanket over" the 'psychic pain' of dysphoria.*

Treating somatoform elaboration in the face of an underlying general medical condition

Very often, clinicians are confronted with patients who suffer from a neurological or other non-psychiatric condition but whose symptoms present as far out of proportion to those expected from their illness. They may also have more intense, more frequent, more atypical, or more functionally disabling symptoms than one would expect.

Patients should undergo a thorough assessment and formulation as described earlier in this text. They should understand that they have two challenges: the first is to optimize the management of their underlying neurological disease (or other non-psychiatric illness). The other challenge is to optimize their emotional health and to work to determine the underlying source of their emotional distress, whether it is a manifestation of their psychological or interpersonal functioning, or due to a psychiatric syndrome associated with their disease.

The therapeutic approach to the somatoform component of the illness should not be different from that used in those patients without evidence of disease. Particular attention should be paid to any emotional factors that were evident at the time of onset of this atypical presentation. For example, a patient with epilepsy may have developed nonepileptic seizures at a time in their life when their epileptic seizures had improved and their medical and social supports consequently decreased. Or a patient with multiple sclerosis may have developed insidious depressive symptoms accompanied by neurological symptoms unexplainable by their disease activity or their disease-modifying medications.

> **Clinical Vignette:** *A 44-year-old woman developed acute-onset dystonia in the context of extreme helplessness when she was unable to access medical care during a cancer scare. Over the years, she developed Parkinson's Disease. She persistently manifested dystonia, but it was only functionally disabling during periods of her life or certain times of the day when she felt particularly helpless or ineffective. Because the disease itself at times rendered her helpless, optimization of her Parkinson's Disease treatment was advocated and arranged as a mandatory part of her Somatoform Disorder treatment, and a behavioural and pharmacological approach to managing fear and helplessness was developed.*

Clinical Vignette: *A 43-year-old accountant had cared for her father during the very difficult end-stage of his Huntington's Disease. She was very familiar with the features of the condition and chose not to have her own genetic testing. At what must have been around her first awareness of subtle signs of the disease, she developed a bizarre gait and flaccid weakness of her legs. This represented a somatoform reaction to her understandable anxiety regarding the diagnosis. She knew that Huntington's did not present with weakness, and the psychogenic symptoms represented both her hope that she did not have the diagnosis, and her underlying distress that she may indeed have the disease.*

Use of electroconvulsive therapy in patients with somatoform disorder

The vast majority of clinicians who work with severely psychiatrically ill individuals will be aware of the controversy around the use of electroconvulsive therapy (ECT). They will also likely have seen the profound positive effect that electroconvulsive therapy can have for individuals with certain conditions such as catatonia or psychosis secondary to a mood disorder. This treatment is best suited to individuals with very definite evidence of profound Axis I psychiatric disturbance that has not responded to months or years of psychological and pharmacological therapies.

We at times use electroconvulsive therapy in individuals with Somatoform Disorders, but only after a great deal of forethought. We have observed a subgroup of individuals who, despite being resistant to all prior therapies, get therapeutic breakthrough with the use of electroconvulsive therapy resulting in greatly improved function. We reported on an open series of 28 such patients, where 22 reported significant improvement after ECT (Leong 2015). There are also some individuals with Somatoform Disorders who have gone on to judicious use of maintenance ECT on an outpatient basis.

As you will recall from prior chapters, the course of a somatoform illness most closely matches the course of the condition that is causing the underlying emotional distress. Some individuals appear to have Somatoform Disorders on the basis of chronic recurrent mood disorders and for some of those individuals, ECT may be a very important part of improving their function in the long run and treating episode recurrence. Thus, the ECT is being used to treat the cause of the underlying dysphoria.

Individuals receiving a series of ECT treatments may experience some post-ECT confusion, more so if they have a greater number of such treatments. During such periods of confusion, for instance 1 to 2 hours after waking from a treatment, some individuals with Somatoform Disorders will show complete resolution of their physical symptoms. This is akin to the resolution one sees in some individuals under the influence of amobarbital or midazolam. In other words, while the individual is confused post-ECT, there is a lack of cognitive resources to produce their physical symptoms. This is again evidence of how Somatoform Disorders are dependent on the patient's belief that they are ill in a particular fashion. The symptoms and signs reconstitute as an individual's confusion lifts. In the same way that narcoanalysis can be used to reveal to an individual that circuitry is intact, video-taping an individual post-ECT (with their prior consent) can also be a useful therapeutic intervention when the video-tape is played to the individual once they are cognitively clear.

Reference:

Leong K, Tham J, Scamvougeras A, Vila-Rodriguez F: Electroconvulsive therapy treatment in patients with somatic symptom and related disorders. Neuropsychiatric Disease and Treatment 2015; 11:2565-2572

CHAPTER SEVEN

FUTURE DIRECTIONS

Education and Understanding

If the general population and health care professionals begin to understand the process of somatization better, those with Somatoform Disorders will be identified more readily and will begin to receive the help they need and deserve. To that end, we would hope that this text will contribute to that spread of knowledge and awareness, and that skills in the assessment and management of these conditions will end up being more widely taught amongst mental health clinicians and primary care providers. We anticipate that internet-based education and debate will be an important part of sharing these concepts more broadly.

Access to Care

Individual health care providers such as psychiatrists, general practitioners, clinical psychologists, physiotherapists, occupational therapists, internists, other medical specialists, and other psychotherapists, are all in a position to use the kind of framework offered in this text to help individuals suffering Somatoform Disorders. Most often 'virtual outpatient teams' are cobbled together ad hoc depending on a patient's needs. The patient may, for example, see a psychiatrist & an occupational therapist, or a clinical psychologist, a GP & a physiotherapist. Thorough liaising takes considerable effort and time on the part of the professionals, and it is a significant challenge to communicate well about complicated and nuanced clinical situations. An ideal solution would be for the creation of multidisciplinary outpatient teams where good and efficient communication is designed into the model, and clinical efforts can be directed most effectively. If one considers the prevalence of Somatoform Disorders, a strong argument can be made that multidisciplinary Somatoform Disorder assessment and treatment centres should be available in all medium to large centres. The high prevalence of these disorders begs for a greater number of health care professionals to become comfortable with assessing and helping this population, and to identify themselves as specializing in this care.

Research

It is usual, towards the end of texts such as this one, for the authors to note that "more research is necessary". We are going to depart a little from making such a blanket statement by saying that some types of research are more necessary than others. We have no doubt that, eventually, Somatoform Disorders will be understood at the molecular level. Any researchers chipping away towards this goal should be applauded, and we will watch any such work with great interest, gleaning anything from discoveries that may be helpful to our patients. Having said that, and despite the impressive recent advances in some aspects of the understanding of neurobiology, we do not expect to see an understanding of Somatoform Disorders at that level in the foreseeable future. Somatoform Disorders are complicated conditions seated in the body's most complex organ. They involve a multitude of brain circuits that are each separately far from being understood. More important research, in our opinion, would be methodologically robust studies looking for the clinical approaches that best help individuals with Somatoform Disorders. A major challenge here is the remarkable heterogeneity of the population. It is likely safe to say that no two patients with Somatoform Disorders are quite alike, and they are often very, very different. It is paramount that researchers keep in mind the two-component nature of the condition in every case - it is no use to attempt to group cohorts by physical symptoms alone, as the underlying sources of dysphoria driving the symptoms are highly likely to be varied across individuals. Thus it would be advisable to use a classification system that takes into account both components in most clinical outcome studies.

Many potential research questions, aimed at furthering understanding and improving clinical outcomes, come to mind:

Do certain prior experiences, attachment styles, or cognitive styles predispose individuals to Somatoform Disorders?

Is it important to attempt to differentiate the form of underlying

dysphoria, or could that be effectively treated with a generic approach?
Other than with regard to types of symptoms, is there a substantial difference between Conversion Disorders and those Somatoform Disorders without functional neurological symptoms?
What clinical features determine good or bad outcome?
Does early treatment influence outcome?
Does identification and treatment of a Somatoform Disorder decrease long term suffering, improve quality of life, and/or reduce need for medical services?
Are mild cases best identified and treated or do they resolve quickly if simply followed?
Can certain features at presentation be used to match patients better with treatments?
Is there a case for using medications, or avoiding medications, early in treatment?
Does very active repeated education regarding the nature of the condition improve outcome?
Which approaches best improve a patient's longterm quality of life?
Would a standardized form of Cognitive Behavioural Therapy (CBT) derived from models such as the one in this book be generalizable and effective?
Is group education and group CBT cost effective?
What patient characteristics may predict benefit from group work?

The Risk of Continuing to Ignore Somatoform Disorders

Early in this text we pointed out the unintentional collusion between patient and clinician that often causes a Somatoform Disorder to be ignored in an individual. This collusion also occurs at the group and community level. The default position, due to a combination of ignorance, stigma, and nihilism, is to continue to behave as though Somatoform Disorders almost don't exist at all (Creed 2006). This position essentially ignores the core plight of the one in four or five patients in primary care waiting-rooms who are there because they are suffering with this kind of condition. Most citizens are completely unaware of the magnitude of the concern.

To change the status quo, considerable effort will be required to educate citizens, medical professionals, and other individuals whose roles may allow them to change things for the better. There will be hurdles - for one, if 'case finding' increases, there may be temporary associated increased health care costs. From our experience with individual cases, these costs often rise temporarily and then, with successful management, fall to rates lower than the initial chronic illness necessitated. This may well be the case at the population level, but that has not yet been conclusively demonstrated. The societal costs of Somatoform Disorders have yet to be carefully studied, but one would imagine that they would be very substantial.

Identifying and helping people with Somatoform Disorder will entail work, it will be inconvenient, it will require effort and resources. None of that should deter us from proceeding to help this population. The truth of the matter is that there are many individuals in the community experiencing this form of complex physical and emotional suffering, and accurate diagnosis and tenacious management will help the majority of them. It is with that in mind that we encourage fellow clinicians, and our communities, to move to actively help people suffering the consequences of Somatoform Disorders.

Reference:

Creed F: Should general psychiatry ignore somatization and hypochondriasis? World Psychiatry 2006; 5:146–150

CHAPTER EIGHT

SUMMARY POINTS

Summary in Point Form of Our Approach to Assessing and Managing Somatoform Disorders

Keep an open mind; avoid premature closure

Therapeutic alliance is paramount

Ensure that you have adequate supportive framework, time, patience, and tenacity to do the necessary work

Be clear regarding the separate phases of the process: assessment, formulation and management

Assessment

Take the time necessary for a thorough assessment

Do not be tempted to partially formulate or commence treatment before you have a diagnosis

Conduct a full assessment:
  Full general medical & psychiatric history
  Physical examination
  Mental status examination
  Investigations as necessary
  Collateral information
  Specialist opinions as necessary

History-taking must be thorough, and as a result is time-intensive

Assess the patient's attribution theories

Listen to the patient's language

Ideally, conduct a thorough physical examination yourself. If this is not possible, liaise with a clinician who can do so

Have a low threshold for obtaining other specialist opinions and second opinions

If you discover general medical disease, arrange for optimal treatment

If physical symptoms and signs are judged, after thorough assessment, to be the result of underlying emotional distress rather than primary physical disease, the patient has a Somatoform Disorder

Make the diagnosis

Use this template to organize your thinking:
'Somatoform Disorder'
1. Physically manifesting as: ____________________
2. Probable cause/s of underlying emotional distress:
   (a) Psychiatric syndrome: ____________________
      As evidenced by: ____________________
   (b) Psychological contributors: ____________________
      As evidenced by: ____________________

Formulation

Schedule a meeting with the patient to share your findings; adequate time, space, and quiet is necessary for this meeting

The patient may elect to have people important to them present - family members, spouse, significant other, or close support

Prepare for the formulation meeting: review all pertinent history, clinical findings, and investigation results very thoroughly

Plan to use the patient's attribution theories and terminology; attempt to meet the patient at any shared area of understanding

Start by validating the severity of the illness, and how profoundly it has interfered with the patient's life

Be thorough in reviewing the patient's story with them

Describe the symptom and sign complex, at length if necessary, integrating an understanding of the course of the illness into that review

Explain the logical steps that you have taken to exclude gross peripheral and demonstrable pathological causes of these symptoms

List the commonly known structural brain pathologies that you have excluded with your assessment

Emphasize how results of any prior assessments and prior investigations have been helpful in synthesizing the current understanding

Share the logical conclusion that the above analysis of their symptoms overwhelmingly indicates that the brain is the seat of the illness

Share your conclusion that the illness is seated in the brain, and that, rather than being caused by clear structural pathology, it is caused by an alteration in the way that the brain is functioning

If appropriate, choose a metaphor or model as a way of understanding and talking about the brain illness, guided by the patient's own concepts regarding the illness: *'Running-interference', 'Neurochemical changes', circuit 'dysregulation', 'Hardware/Software', 'Switchboard', Phantom limb, Referred pain*

'Vicious cycle' idea may be applicable, where central brain dysfunction sets up actual changes in periphery, such as muscle bracing, that then perpetuate the peripheral symptoms

The conclusions from the assessment means that a definitive diagnosis can now be made

Give the condition a name: it is a 'Somatoform Disorder', a condition where brain-based distress is indirectly, involuntarily, and unconsciously, expressed as physical symptoms

Patients who have shown developing insight into the role of 'stress' or emotion in their illness may benefit from discussion of 'brain-based emotional distress'

If appropriate, discuss the underlying process of 'somatization', the involuntary physical expression of emotional distress. Some may be ready to entertain emotional distress as a causative factor, others not

Emphasize that the process is unconscious and involuntary

Share that these conditions are relatively common

Discuss the lack of complete 100% diagnostic certainty

Reassure regarding a plan for ongoing monitoring for any sign of sinister general medical disease

Validate the veracity of the illness: the condition is as 'real' as any other form of medical condition

If appropriate, discuss other terminology used to describe somatoform conditions, such as 'Conversion Disorder', 'Somatoform Pain', 'Somatic Symptom Disorders', 'functional disorders', and, even, 'hysteria'

You may actively encourage some patients to do their own reading about their condition; invite them to bring any articles or ideas that they may want to discuss

Address any perceived delay in diagnosis: this is not unusual in complex conditions

Express unity with past clinicians, as appropriate

Emphasize that the condition is treatable

If possible and appropriate, share what you understand of the nature of the underlying emotional distress

Emphasize that the mechanisms are unconscious and involuntary, and that you know they are not malingering

Address the common "Nothing is wrong/All in my head" concerns

Reinforce that the illness is not consciously caused, but the patient's efforts will benefit them in recovery

Again, validate prior suffering, and share an understanding of how the patient has attempted to overcome their illness

Be prepared to support patients who may have a dysphoric response to your formulation, which challenges their ego-defences and, in some cases, longstanding patterns of illness behaviour (review pp. 80-81, 'The Formulation That Feels Overly Intrusive')

Frame a path to recovery; the patient has the ability to conquer the illness

Suggest a second formulation meeting; encourage the patient to bring any questions or thoughts that arise to that meeting; suggest they jot down any important questions that arise

Meet again to answer questions and reiterate the major points of understanding

Encourage the patient to involve their partner, family, caregivers, or other support in one of the meetings; share the major points again in that context

Be a supportive advocate for your patient

Allow the patient time to consider their options

If the patient decides to proceed with recommended treatment, proceed to the management phase

Management

Customize treatment to each patient

Aim is to achieve resolution of physical symptoms and treat underlying emotional distress & other manifestations of psychiatric illness

Always keep in mind that there are two main components of the condition: the emotional distress and the physical manifestations

You will simultaneously be considering and using:
Psychological and behavioural interventions,
Pharmacological and other biological interventions, and
Physical therapies targeting psychogenic symptoms and general conditioning

Help the individual with similar techniques to those which you would utilize when helping other patients with similar types of emotional distress

If the distress appears to be more the result of psychological processes, make more use of psychotherapeutic techniques

If the patient has clear evidence of psychopathology related to an endogenous psychiatric disorder, with neurovegetative changes, medications are likely indicated

Judicious use of medications targeting, for instance, sleep disturbance, excessive anxiety, or depressive symptoms may result in improved capacity to make use of psychotherapeutic techniques

Regardless of cause of distress, ongoing educational, supportive, cognitive and behavioural psychotherapeutic techniques will be useful for complete recovery

Develop a stepwise, flexible plan for each patient

The aim of management is to improve the individual's overall quality of life

Psychological work is customized to patient and clinician factors: use techniques that make sense to you, and that you have found to be helpful for other patients with similar forms of emotional distress

Take into account the patient's attribution theories and world view, and their education, intellect, and degree of insight

Behavioural interventions regarding daily structure, exercise and sleep are often helpful

A psychodynamic understanding of the patient will often inform the way in which one directs therapies, but a purely psychodynamic approach to treatment is not recommended, particularly early in the therapy

Continue to emphasize and reiterate the understanding of the condition

For some patients, the concept of 'stress' affecting the brain is helpful; in others a mechanistic discussion of neurotransmitters and dysregulated circuits affecting motor or sensory circuits may make most sense

The cognitive framework for understanding the condition, presented in the formulation, and shaped over time with the patient such that it makes sense to both the patient and the treating clinician, is the core model to which you return during the period of treatment

The understanding of the patient and their condition may change over time; be prepared for that.

The initial impression about the underlying cause of the patient's emotional distress may prove to be inaccurate: further history or new clinical evidence may emerge

Keep the 'basket' of symptoms together: frequently reiterate all symptoms that are targets of treatment

Emphasize that the central physical symptom is not the only target of treatment: the goal is good overall recovery

Enhance patient motivation as it is a major factor in determining positive outcome

Target complete resolution of physical symptoms

Prepare the patient for changes in physical symptoms; temporarily physical symptoms may be exacerbated with the commencement of more active management approaches

Encourage the patient's development of insight

As somatic defences fall away and physical symptoms improve, do not be surprised by the emergence of more obvious psychiatric syndromes; Treat these as you would similar symptoms in any other patient

Assist the patient in understanding what may for them be frighteningly overt emotional distress; Explain it in terms of the overall model

Specific couple or family work may be particularly helpful in situations where it is determined that psychological distress and interpersonal functioning is an important part of the engine driving the somatoform condition

Use of medications is determined by features suggesting a neurobiological pathophysiology to the underlying emotional distress

Suggest medications where careful analysis leads you to believe that the potential benefit of a medication significantly outweighs the risks of a trial of that medication

Understand the reluctance of many patients to use medications; counsel them thoroughly about the risks and benefits; suggest they see medications as "useful tools"

Employ a stepwise, symptom-driven approach to the use of medications: a journey to find a good fit between the patient and a straight-forward medication regimen that works

The choice of medication is based on the constellation of psychiatric and psychological symptoms and signs: the clinician should use medications with which they are familiar, and which they would use for a similar constellation of psychiatric symptoms in other settings

When the condition is more treatment resistant, and where there is evidence of underlying psychosis, OCD, or severe mood instability, some patients may benefit from dopamine-blockers

Narcoanalysis can be useful for diagnosis and treatment

Optimize medications previously instituted for presumed somatic indications; wean patients off these whenever possible, especially from opiates

All biological therapies are used in the context of ongoing psychological work

Target general 'reconditioning', and start an activity schedule

Physiotherapy, or various other forms of direct physical therapies, should be used to specifically focus on somatoform symptoms; the aim is complete recovery of physical function

Even though not the primary intention, the supportive emotional effects of 'hands-on' therapies such as physiotherapy and massage can play a role in 'mobilizing' the physical and the psychological factors inhibiting physical function

While physical therapies are being actively used, prepare the individual for possible substantial breakthroughs in physical symptoms; let the patient know that it would not be unusual for them to suddenly improve

Broad Principles

An effective therapeutic alliance is central to successful outcome

Be prepared for ongoing care

Positively reinforce improvement; frame gains in functioning as victories for the patient

Be a sensible advocate on behalf of the patient, within their family, social and occupational domains

The patient's personal internal motivation will correlate very highly with a positive outcome; support the patient while at the same time assisting them in developing independent strength

Let the patient lead the way

Allow the patient space and time with regard to return to their occupation

Address any apparent anger or blame regarding the course of the condition, including frustration at medical professionals; 'the villain is the illness'

In most medical systems, a 'virtual' outpatient multidisciplinary team is patched together for each patient, depending on their needs

If working with a multidisciplinary team, ensure good communication

Prognosis is most closely related to the prognosis of the underlying cause of the emotional distress, less so to the physical manifestations

Biological and psychological factors are of equal importance

Attempt to thoroughly understand the patient's beliefs about their condition

Exploration and comprehension of the patient's values and world view, of their cultural and religious perspectives, will be invaluable when it comes to assisting them with their recovery

Be prepared for complex countertransference in some instances

Clinicians will differ in their specific approaches to the treatment of the underlying emotional distress

Aim for complete resolution of physical symptoms, and optimal treatment of underlying emotional distress

Be tenacious

ON THE CLASSIFICATION OF SOMATOFORM DISORDERS

Truth is the daughter of time, not of authority.
- Francis Bacon, essayist

Classification reflects understanding

It is a great challenge to classify medical disorders in instances where we do not yet have a clear understanding of the underlying genetics and pathophysiology. Without molecular or tissue information, we are forced to attempt to classify the disorder at the symptom and sign level in the hope that the entity thus defined ends up representing a valid disease. The success of such a syndromal classification system is ultimately dependent on whether it ends up being generally consistent with the as yet unknown underlying mechanisms of the condition or conditions. To put this another way, one is hoping that subdividing the population according to patterns of signs and symptoms at a clinical level will also subdivide the population in a meaningful fashion at the pathophysiological and genetic/causation level.

The features of a valid syndrome (Robins & Guze 1970) are that it would reflect a true underlying causative & pathophysiological process, that there are demonstrable boundaries between it and other conditions, and that it would demonstrate stability over the course of the condition. The more pathophysiologically valid a clinical syndrome, the more reliable and stable the resultant diagnoses, and the more useful and generalizable any conclusions drawn about the management of the syndrome.

Somatoform Disorders, conditions where emotional distress is expressed indirectly as physical symptoms through a process called 'somatization', have long been referred to in different ways and by different names. There are some excellent accounts in the literature of the history of the understanding and naming of these conditions. The review by Lipowski (1988) is to be recommended, as well as the more recent accounts by Trimble & Reynolds (2016) and Stone (2016). For the sake of context, we will briefly summarize some of the relevant older ideas about these conditions before discussing recent classification struggles in greater detail.

Historical perspective

Three thousand years ago the Egyptians, and then later the Greeks, described syndromes with physical and emotional symptoms that were (notoriously, by our current sensibilities) attributed to pathologies of the uterus. This gave the name 'hysteria' to these conditions. In the 1600's Sydenham described physical and mental symptoms of hysteria and hypochondriasis, seeing each as "disturbance and inconsistency both of the mind and the body". Sims in the 1700's distinguished hysteria, hypochondriasis and melancholia. Both Sydenham and Sims, when describing hysteria, emphasized the presence of symptoms of depression and anxiety along with physical symptoms (Lipowski 1988).

In 1859 Briquet described a syndrome where individuals had lifelong, multitudinous physical symptoms without apparent physical disease. He saw the brain as mediating these symptoms (Mai 1980). This syndrome, with some further shaping, developed into the 'somatization disorder' used in classification systems up until very recently. Charcot emphasized the hereditary nature of hysteria and showed that he could induce symptoms with hypnosis. Freud and Breuer developed theories that the symptoms of hysteria were acting as an ego defence, with physical symptoms emerging to decrease intrapsychic dysphoria. In the early 1900's, the term 'somatization' was first used, with Menninger describing somatization reactions as "visceral expressions of anxiety which is thereby prevented from being conscious" (Lipowski 1988).

In the twentieth century it became apparent that there were major challenges in this area with regard to reliability of diagnosis. Movement towards better defining and classifying these syndromes began. In one landmark study, sixty-six women who had been given a diagnosis of 'hysteria' between 1927 and 1932 were reassessed 22 to 25 years later; it was found that their clinical course had varied a great deal. In fact, 1 in 3 had developed psychotic illness. It was noted that the original criteria had been "variable and under defined" and authors of that study saw a need for a greater precision in diagnosing what was at that time still called 'hysteria' (Ziegler & Paul 1954). A retrospective chart study and followup published in 1962 (Perley & Guze) defined a syndrome of hysteria closely related to the principles suggested by Briquet in the 1800's. The authors found that 90% of 28 patients with a diagnosis of or suggestive of hysteria still met criteria at 6 to 8 year follow-up. Those criteria included dramatic or complicated medical histories starting prior to the age of 35 and a minimum of 15 symptoms distributed among at least 9 of 10 groups of symptoms. The groupings did not show much face validity. For example, one group of symptoms included 'fatigue, lump in throat, fainting spells, visual blurring, weakness or dysuria'. The authors concluded that the criteria "define a valid and distinct clinical syndrome". It should be noted that the syndrome thus described represented patients with multiple symptoms and severe disorder.

Enter DSM Somatoform Disorders

In 1980, the American Psychiatric Association's 'Diagnostic and Statistical Manual of Mental Disorders' ('DSM'), in its third edition (DSM-III), discarded the term 'hysteria' and introduced the category 'Somatoform Disorders', a group of syndromes with the presence of "physical symptoms suggesting physical disorder". DSM-III used subcategories of Somatization Disorder, Conversion Disorder, Psychogenic Pain Disorder and Hypochondriasis within the Somatoform category (APA 1980).

It is impossible to discuss the classification of any complex neurobehavioural condition without giving special consideration to the ubiquitous DSM. There are many legitimate criticisms that can be levelled against the DSM. It is fair to note that some categories and subcategories of the DSM are shaped with limited empiric support, low reliability, and may include contradictory elements. There is also valid discussion regarding the DSM's possible over-pathologization of common aspects of human existence (Davis 1997, Frances 2013), as well as its arguable cultural 'U.S.-centricity'. There is also a need for very serious considerations of conflict regarding industry influence (both 'pharma' and insurers), and the related fact that the American Psychiatric Association profits grandly from the existence of the DSM in its current form (Frances 2012). Further, there is valid concern that some decisions that shape the DSM reflect administrative or political expedience rather than what should be the paramount goal: to describe valid syndromes. Such has been the divisiveness and tenacity of the debate that after the publication of DSM-5 in 2013, more than one mental health care professional has opined "there will never be a DSM-6".

Challenging times for psychiatry

In parallel with criticisms of the DSM, there has been something of a slow-motion multi-decade crisis in psychiatry, as the early promises of the 1980's, in fields such as neurogenetics and functional neuroimaging, have as yet failed to translate into any appreciable gains for people suffering from psychiatric conditions. There is a strong argument to be made that unrealistic expectations and the instillation of false hope have hobbled the field. One can point to many mainstream news articles announcing the 'discovery' of 'a gene', or some other 'breakthrough' for one or another psychiatric disorder, the articles each invariably ending with hope that this would translate into benefit for citizens with the relevant disorder. These articles manifest when researchers seeking publicity and funding meet journalists seeking a story. The unfortunate result is a public that is understandably jaded by decades of unrealistic claims and projections. This justifiable skeptical mood has been compounded by the recent wave of findings that various forms of bias exaggerated the initial reported efficacy of some psychotropic medications, such as the antidepressants. Partly as a consequence of the resultant frustration, increasing doubts are being expressed about specific methods such as syndromal classification and even about the scientific method itself. Witness the increasing favour given to 'qualitative' research, an approach that may entail useful exploratory endeavours, but which is not a replacement for the rigorous testing of hypotheses in quantitative work.

The core truth here is that the brain is a very, very complex organ. The pathophysiologies affecting it are multiple and complicated, and it is going to take humankind many, many decades to tease apart all of these mysteries at the molecular level. The neurobiology of complex neuropsychiatric conditions is complex (repetition intended). This is simply the truth of it, and pretending otherwise will doom us to years of maldirected endeavours and even more disappointments.

But there is a risk that the proverbial baby gets thrown out with the bathwater. The fact that DSM-5 uses a syndromal approach, and the fact that progress has not been rapid in the understanding or management of many disorders, are not arguments against a DSM-like approach. It is not that the DSM "hasn't worked" but rather that the aforementioned unrealistic expectations have weighed on the DSM, and indeed on the whole of psychiatry as a field. Shaping and improving syndromal diagnostic systems is the best, and indeed the only way forward for the field. Good syndromal diagnostic systems will offer a framework around which we can eventually, many years hence, more fully understand the neurobiology of these complex conditions, and the doubtlessly even more complex ways in which the neurobiology interacts with the environment. The syndromal systems used may take the form of the existing DSM or ICD (International Statistical Classification of Diseases and Related Health Problems (WHO 1992)). We can also see a strong argument for the development of a non-proprietary open-source syndromal diagnostic system, with no hurdles to the free sharing of scientific ideas and information. In contrast, for one to simply print the DSM-5 'Somatic Symptom Disorder' criteria here for the purpose of discussion, one would have to go through an application process that would take weeks and would ultimately depend on permission being granted by the APA (APA 2018). We would rather advocate for clinicians and researchers around the globe to be using a way of understanding and classifying mental health conditions that belongs to no single entity.

DSM-IV suffered problems

DSM-IV, published in 1994, dealt with Somatoform Disorders by describing a group of symptoms that had in common the "presence of physical symptoms that suggest a general medical condition" that were "not fully explained by a general medical condition". This group of syndromes included 'Somatization Disorder' which was a severe form of Somatoform Disorder defined by having a duration of many years and requiring eight symptoms across four groups. 'Undifferentiated Somatoform Disorder', however, was a far less severe condition requiring only one symptom and 6 months duration to meet criteria. 'Conversion

Disorder', characterized by symptoms suggesting neurological illness, crucially required that the clinician judge psychological factors or stressors to be instrumental in the cause of the illness. Similarly, the surprisingly non-specifically named 'Pain Disorder' required a judgement regarding the importance of psychological factors. 'Hypochondriasis', 'Body Dysmorphic Disorder' and 'Somatoform Disorder Not Otherwise Specified' were the other syndromes in this category. In addition, elsewhere in DSM-IV, there were other syndromes where physical symptoms were central, examples being 'Delusional Disorder Somatic Subtype', 'Psychological Factors Affecting Medical Condition', 'Factitious Disorder' and 'Malingering'.

There were significant limitations in the way that DSM-IV classified Somatoform Disorders. One major concern was the unclear basis for separating the syndromes. For instance, similar sets of physical symptoms, without underlying general medical cause, could exist across Somatization Disorder, Undifferentiated Somatoform Disorder, Conversion Disorder, Hypochondriasis, Body Dysmorphic Disorder and Delusional Disorder Somatic Subtype. There was a strong argument to be made that some of these conditions were more similar than different.

Furthermore, there were significant threshold and sensitivity problems. In a study looking at 119 patients in family practitioner waiting rooms, Somatization Disorder criteria were met in just one patient, whereas as many as 94 met criteria for Undifferentiated Somatoform Disorder (Lynch 1999). Other studies confirmed that DSM-IV Somatization Disorder itself had a very low prevalence (estimated 0.4 %) (Creed 2004). Thus it appeared that criteria were too tight for one diagnostic entity and too loose for the other, with neither serving as a useful instrument for separating the majority of individuals with significant somatoform symptoms from the general population.

There was also strong evidence that clinicians simply weren't using the DSM-IV Somatoform Disorder classification system. Although known to be prevalent, these disorders were severely under-diagnosed by clinicians in the field. For instance, of the 28 million 'Wellpoint/Anthem Blue Cross' members who had clinical encounters in 2008, only 0.04% received a primary diagnosis of a Somatoform Disorder (Levenson 2011).

DSM-IV did not promote a clinically useful understanding of somatoform concepts and it likely discouraged clinicians from identifying these disorders. A 2009 survey of physicians revealed that the definition of Somatoform Disorders and its subgroups was unclear to many (Dimsdale 2011). A clinician's lack of clarity, along with a patient's poor insight (an integral component of the unconscious somatoform process), leads to an unintended collaboration that results in the avoidance of the recognition of these disorders. Under DSM-IV, most individuals suffering a Somatoform Disorder did not get identified as such. Further, the poor state of affairs resulted in the category being left off most national surveys of mental health, and almost certainly made research in the field less attractive (Creed 2006).

The crux of the matter was that DSM-IV did not classify Somatoform Disorders in a valid fashion, and thus, there was little or nothing to be gained from using it clinically, or from a research perspective. The category was clearly in need of an overhaul.

The development of DSM-5

The DSM-5 Working Group, charged with developing a new category to replace DSM-IV's Somatoform Disorders, consisted of ten specialists in the field (8 MDs, 2 PhDs; 6 from the US, 2 from the UK, 1 from Hong Kong, and 1 from Canada), most of whom worked to this purpose from about 2000 until publication of DSM-5 in 2013.

Through these years, the classification of these disorders was much debated in the literature. The main areas of discussion were the wisdom of using 'medically unexplained symptoms' as part of the criteria, the validity of subdivisions, and the nomenclature. Some argued for a fundamental change in the category (Sharpe & Carson 2001, Rief 2004, Mayou 2005, Kroenke 2006); others for essentially retaining the 'somatoform' concept even if making other refinements (Fink 2005, De Gucht 2006, Hiller 2006, Levenson 2006). The authors of this text, along with six of their colleagues, wrote a letter to the working group responding to their April 18 2011 'Justification of Criteria-Somatic Symptoms' draft (APA 2011). Discussion and feedback had been invited, and we laid out our critique of the intended changes (Scamvougeras 2011). That letter is reproduced in this book (Appendix VI: Letter to DSM-5 Working Group, pp. 195-202).

DSM-5 represents very substantial changes to the way in which these disorders are understood and classified, changes that have profound clinical and research implications. DSM-5 "reconceptualized" Somatoform Disorders, changing the category name to 'Somatic Symptom and Related Disorders', a group of disorders all characterized by the presence of physical symptoms. The most profound change within this new category was the creation of a newly defined core disorder, 'Somatic Symptom Disorder' (SSD), a syndrome characterized by persistent and clinically significant somatic complaints accompanied by excessive and disproportionate health-related thoughts, feelings, and behaviours regarding the physical symptoms. Patients meeting DSM-IV criteria for Somatization Disorder, Undifferentiated Somatoform Disorder, and Pain Disorder would now very likely all meet SSD criteria. But, SSD would now also include individuals *with demonstrable physical disease* with "excessive thoughts, feelings or behaviours" about their physical symptoms, because, crucially, there is *no longer any need for symptoms to be 'medically unexplained'*. Further, SSD now ends up including the majority of individuals previously diagnosed with 'Hypochondriasis' (DSM-5, p. 311).

Conversion Disorder remains a separate condition under DSM-5, gaining the new co-title 'Functional Neurological Symptom Disorder' (FNSD). Here the clinician judges that "clinical findings provide evidence of incompatibility between the symptom and recognized neurological or medical conditions". In other words, the symptoms are 'medically unexplained', so the need to make that distinction is retained for a diagnosis of Conversion Disorder/FNSD. But there is no longer the need to determine that "psychological factors are judged to be associated" (as was the case in DSM-IV), nor does the diagnosis require the clinician to deem that the symptoms are not consciously feigned.

So, the crux of the change in DSM-5 was the move away from a disorder or disorders characterized by 'medically unexplained symptoms' (MUS), towards conditions where physical symptoms caused 'excessive thoughts, feelings or behaviours' whether medically explained or not. Even though Conversion Disorder/FNSD retains the 'medically unexplained' component, the loss of the need for that judgement for non-neurological functional symptoms and signs (for symptoms such as fatigue or pain) represents a marked move away from defining what the authors consider 'Somatoform Disorders'. The change in nomenclature, and to a certain extent, the collapse of subdivisions of disorder, are all changes that are more secondary when compared with the importance of the move away from 'medically unexplained symptoms' (MUS).

The reasons for the fundamental changes in the classification of these conditions were shared with the public, both during the development process (APA 2011), and on publication of DSM-5 (Dimsdale 2013).

The DSM-5 rationale for the eradication of 'medically unexplained symptoms' as a central idea in these disorders
(*rationale in italics*, our responses in regular text):

"*The reliability of assessing whether or not there is an explanation for somatic symptoms is notoriously poor*" (Dimsdale 2013).
In actual fact, after a thorough clinical assessment including special investigations as necessary, a clinician can draw the conclusion that symptoms are 'medically unexplained' with a similar degree of certainty as one would have in making the diagnosis in many general medical conditions and other psychiatric diagnoses (see Appendix II: Risk of Misdiagnosis pp. 161-3). Thorough clinical assessment, with the diagnostic tools available to us, allow clinicians to make such judgments at an acceptable level of accuracy.

"*..some MUS are not so much 'Unexplained' as 'Unexamined'*" (Dimsdale 2013).
This is a criticism of incomplete assessment, not of the concept of drawing the conclusion that symptoms are medically unexplained. This same criticism could be made in the case of any other psychiatric or general medical condition. A thorough assessment is always essential before making a diagnosis of a Somatoform Disorder.

"*A diagnosis built upon a foundation of MUS is perilous because it reinforces mind/body dualism.*" (Dimsdale 2013).
It is thereby argued that to say that physical symptoms are 'medically unexplained' may lead some patients and clinicians to conclude that the mind and body are distinct and separable, and that the physical symptoms may be due to some 'non-physical' process. This dualistic thinking is incorrect. All neuropsychiatric conditions are mediated by brain function. All aspects of Somatoform Disorders are products of complex brain function and dysfunction, the specific nature of which

we do not yet understand. It is vital that we address the challenge presented by any tendency to dualistic thinking head-on. The answer is not to abandon the concept of Somatoform Disorders out of fear that some may misunderstand, but rather to wrestle with the challenge, to engage the field in discussion, and to educate clinicians and patients about the nature of these conditions. They do indeed involve complex interactions between what most of us would consider to be the mind and the body. But all of these interactions are manifestations of various levels of biological brain/body function. A thorough understanding of the somatoform process may even serve as an integrative force, and prove to be supportive of arguments against dualism.

"*...the MUS approach is not well accepted by patients who feel that MUS implies that their symptoms are inauthentic and "all in your head". This is a poor basis for a therapeutic alliance with patients who are suffering distressing somatic complaints.*" (Dimsdale 2013)
A similar challenge exists when helping all individuals suffering other psychiatric and psychological conditions. This challenge is partly related to the stigma regarding mental illness that persists in our society, and partly due to the complex emotions (including fear, puzzlement, guilt, anger) that an individual may experience when they have the thought that something may be awry with their mind. The only way forward is to understand these conditions for what they are, and on the foundation of thorough assessment and empathic therapeutic alliance, to help those suffering from them. A clinician should, in a supportive fashion, share the truth about the condition with the patient. These disorders are, indeed, all mediated by brain function and dysfunction, so they are indeed *literally* based in large part "in one's head"; however, from a *figurative* perspective they are *not* "imagined"... so this distinction must be made clear for the patient. The unconscious and involuntary nature of the somatization process must be emphasized, and the nature of the condition plainly described. To avoid the truth because it may be unpalatable does not serve patients well at all, as optimal management is predicated on a valid understanding of the disorder. It is also poor science.

"*It bases a diagnosis on a negative...*" (APA 2011).
"*... a medical diagnosis does not usually define a disorder based on the absence of something*" (Dimsdale 2013).
Clinicians go through a logical process of elimination whenever they

consider the differential diagnosis for any set of symptoms and signs. Exclusion of known diseases is part of every diagnostic process. If, at the end of such a process, the clinical picture suggests 'medically unexplained symptoms', then they should be called that. That judgment is not qualitatively very different from what we are doing with many other disease entities. It is further implied in the DSM-5 discussion that making the diagnosis of a MUS is somehow a 'negative' step in a broader sense, in that clinicians and patients see it as the 'taking away' of something rather than a 'positive' diagnosis. Many diagnoses in general medicine embrace the fact that there are unknown components to the pathogenesis. For instance, after ruling out hypertension secondary to renal, endocrine, or other general medical conditions, the hypertension is labeled 'idiopathic'. Patients don't complain that they have lost something or had something 'taken away' in that process. We would argue that making a 'Somatoform Disorder' diagnosis is as proactive a diagnostic step as the making of any other diagnosis, and we believe that we in the field should work to actively frame it as such. The patient should be informed that their syndrome is the result of complex brain and mind processes, not demonstrable brain or peripheral tissue pathology. This has positive implications for treatment, and we help the patient understand that. Indeed, we would suggest that it is the clinician's *duty* to make such judgments and to offer to treat the patient accordingly. It is only with such a judgment call that the disorder can be understood, and appropriate management instituted.

The DSM-5 rationale for the change in nomenclature from 'Somatoform Disorders' to 'Somatic Symptom and Related Disorders'

With the move away from 'medically unexplained symptoms', it is not surprising that DSM-5 moved away from the 'somatoform' label. Nevertheless, an additional set of reasons was offered for removing the term, namely: it *"has been difficult to understand"*, it was *"a neologism, blending Latin and Greek"*, and because it was *"often confused with somatization disorder"* (Dimsdale 2013). Various terms have been suggested as the best label to refer to the group of conditions based on 'medically unexplained symptoms', including 'functional', 'psychogenic', 'psychosomatic', 'psychophysiological', 'somatic', 'somatization' and 'somatoform'. We argue that 'somatoform' is precisely the word that most elegantly captures the very essence of these conditions. It suggests that an illness is 'in the form of' the body, while at the very same time implying that there is more to it than that. The fact that 'somatoform' is a Greek-Latin hybrid does not in any way detract from its possible use, but rather puts it in the good company of many other such hybrid medical words that we use every day: neuroscience, neurotransmitter, antacid, diverticulosis, hemoglobin, hypertension, intradermal, neutrophil, retinopathy, tuberculosis; - all examples of Latin-Greek hybrids (Dirckx 1977). 'Somatoform' has no more potential for being confused with 'somatization' than does 'somatic symptom'. This is a matter of educating clinicians and patients, and being clear and consistent in our use of the term.

Of course, nomenclature should be closely and logically tied to the nature of the condition to which it is being applied. As DSM-5 represented a wholesale change in the conceptualization of this group of conditions, one could argue that the new nomenclature better suits the newly defined condition. However, the new DSM-5 nomenclature is still problematic. The broad category itself should more completely be called 'Somatic Symptom Disorders and Related Disorders' but for the sake of brevity (one would imagine), it was shortened to 'Somatic Symptom and Related Disorders'. This was a mistake, as this is an inelegant and ambiguous category name (is there a condition called 'Somatic Symptom'?). Further, considering the specific 'Somatic Symptom Disorder' label: this is arguably a far more confusing term than any of those using the term 'somatoform' because on the face of it, it could easily be misunderstood to describe *any* disorder that involves a physical ('somatic') symptom. In this sense it is potentially hobbled by its lack of specificity and its breadth, as was 'Pain Disorder' in DSM-IV.

The collapse of subdivisions that had no validity in DSM-IV into a single diagnostic entity

The collapsing of DSM-IV Somatization Disorder, Undifferentiated Somatoform Disorder and Pain Disorder into a single continuum or entity makes excellent sense. We would applaud this development if it were happening under a 'somatoform' umbrella. In fact, we would argue that there is a place for going further, by including Conversion Disorder along with other somatoform conditions into a single somatoform diagnostic entity or continuum. Granted, some pseudoneurological symptoms can be more definitively demonstrated to be medically unexplained, but we know that symptoms affecting "voluntary motor or sensory function" are not materially different in underlying mechanism, or in any other consistent way, from other somatoform symptoms such as psychogenic pain, fatigue, sense of bloating, palpitations, or dizziness, that likewise do not follow patterns of demonstrative disease. These symptoms co-occur in Somatoform Disorder patients, and resolve with the same therapeutic approaches. We do not believe there is a valid distinction between the syndrome of Conversion Disorder and the syndrome of non-neurological Somatoform Disorders. They are simply different expressions of the same underlying phenomenon. We would thus argue that the collapse of DSM-IV subgroups makes good sense, but not under the current DSM-5 conceptualization.

Logical and linguistic inconsistencies within SSD criteria

Aside from the central disagreements that we have regarding the change in nomenclature and the broadening of the central concept, there are also some more peripheral, but still important, problems with the Somatic Symptom Disorder (SSD) diagnostic criteria.

The SSD criteria contain within them logical inconsistencies:

The C criteria requires that, to qualify for a diagnosis of SSD, "*the state of being symptomatic is persistent (typically more than 6 months).*"

If the patient meets the A, B and C criteria, there are then three 'Specifiers', the second of which states: "*Specify if: Persistent: A persistent course is characterized by severe symptoms, marked impairment, and long duration (more than 6 months).*" Basic logic applied by someone with no knowledge of this specific condition, or even, for that matter, of psychiatry, reveals inconsistencies and contradictions in those two diagnostic items. For the diagnosis to be made, the condition already has to have persisted for more than 6 months, so then considering again whether it is 'persistent' for 'more than 6 months' is redundant and makes no sense. Furthermore, the specifier contains poor use of language and internal contradictions - judging whether a condition is 'persistent' is, in this context, all about *duration* and has nothing to do with either 'severity' or 'impairment', so why are these considerations introduced here under this specifier? Such details are important in diagnostic criteria, where clarity and lack of ambiguity are desirable features.

Overall, the DSM-5 Working Group argued that the core problems with DSM-IV Somatoform Disorders were based on confusing nomenclature, and numerous untenable problems relating to identifying 'medically unexplained symptoms'. We would disagree: the problem with DSM-IV was not the 'somatoform' name, nor the concept itself, but rather the fact that the classification system did not promote a clear understanding of somatoform conditions, and the main disorders did not identify and separate out patients with Somatoform Disorders in a clinically useful or valid fashion. Thus the system was hardly used, and under it the majority of individuals with Somatoform Disorders were not identified or assisted.

The crucial difference between the approach of DSM-5 and the approach for which we advocate is around the clinician's judgment regarding medically unexplained symptoms. DSM-5 and others are advocating for "*acceptance of etiological neutrality about those symptoms that are not clearly associated with a general medical condition*" (Mayou 2005). One can see the attraction of the apparent logical rigour and prudence suggested by the DSM-5 approach: How can we ever be 100% sure that there is not some as-yet-unidentified medical condition causing the symptoms and signs? And, as we can't be 100% certain, let us rather withhold judgement. But diagnoses in complex neurobehavioural conditions are seldom made with certainty. In making judgment calls about 'medically unexplained symptoms' and the nature of Somatoform Disorders, the clinician has to weigh the risk of error in diagnosis *against the risk of not making a diagnosis where one can reasonably be made.* The risks of not making a diagnosis include potentially treatable illnesses not being treated. Forgoing distinguishing 'medically unexplained symptoms' will lump a group of potentially treatable or even curable individuals (those with Somatoform Disorders) in with a group who are going to be encouraged to "learn to live with their illness" (individuals with demonstrable illness and excessive distress about symptoms). This, we would argue, does not serve the vast majority of these patients well.

One would hope that subsequent classification systems would avoid the pitfalls of DSM-5 Somatic Symptom Disorder. Unfortunately, ICD 11 is in actual fact following the path of DSM-5 SSD with the introduction of 'Bodily Distress Disorder', characterized by "*the presence of bodily symptoms that are distressing to the individual and excessive attention directed toward the symptoms, which may be manifest by repeated contact with health care providers*" (WHO 2018, Gureje 2016).

A suggested classification system

We would argue for ongoing use of the clinician's judgment regarding 'medically unexplained symptoms' and the resultant 'somatoform' concept. We believe that this distinction defines a discrete syndrome that will ultimately prove to be a valid disorder or group of disorders.

Further, as there is no discernible etiological reason to separate somatoform presentations on the basis of whether the symptoms appear neurological or not, we would suggest the collapse of all somatoform syndromes (including conversion-type syndromes) into a single 'Somatoform Disorder' entity.

We would suggest the use of a classification system (see below) that is structured to strongly emphasize, and be a constant reminder of, the dual nature of somatoform conditions. Each individual with a 'Somatoform Disorder' has two components to their illness: the physical manifestation (the psychogenic symptoms and signs) and the underlying distress (the 'engine' of the illness).

The suggested system (see also pp. 25-31) is related to approaches suggested by others in that it is primarily descriptive (Hiller 2006) and uses some aspects of multidimensional approaches (Sharpe 1995, De Gucht 2006). It differs in that it is less purely empirical, and its structure reflects our understanding of underlying mechanisms. Thus we would predict it will be more helpful for clinicians and patients, and at the same time be a sound foundation for research aimed at better understanding of the conditions.

Suggested Diagnostic Template:

'Somatoform Disorder'
(present if apparent physical symptoms and signs are judged, after thorough assessment, to be the result of underlying emotional distress rather than primary physical disease)

1. **Physically manifesting as:** ______________________
   (list and describe all of the physical somatoform symptoms and signs)

2. **Probable cause/s of underlying emotional distress:**

(a) **Psychiatric syndrome:** ____________________
As evidenced by: ____________________
(list psychiatric symptoms and signs, including those pertaining to mood, anxiety, thought form, thought content, attention, motivation, perception, behaviour; as well as neurovegetative features such as sleep disturbance, appetite change, weight change, low energy/fatigue, decreased libido, psychomotor agitation/slowing.)

(b) **Psychological contributors:** ____________________
As evidenced by: ____________________
(psychological features including developmental factors, personality, coping style, conflicts, current circumstances, current stressors.)

So the template looks like this:
'Somatoform Disorder'
1. Physically manifesting as: ____________________
2. Probable cause/s of underlying emotional distress:
(a) Psychiatric syndrome: ____________________
As evidenced by: ____________________
(b) Psychological contributors: ____________________
As evidenced by: ____________________

The framework as presented is clinically useful. It clarifies the clinician's understanding at time of diagnosis, and it can be used to follow progress through serial assessments and management.

Under this classification system, in a clinical setting, any patient presenting with somatoform symptoms has a Somatoform Disorder. For research purposes, one would have to further operationalize the description of the condition with attention to features such as threshold at which the diagnosis is made, ways of assessing severity & degree of disability, and duration of the condition. As we have emphasized before, it would be important in research studies to keep in mind the dual nature of the condition, ideally grouping individuals who have similar underlying causes of distress and similar physical manifestations. If that proves to be too much of a methodological challenge, it would make more sense to group by pattern of underlying emotional distress rather than by physical manifestations.

References:

American Psychiatric Association: Diagnostic and statistical manual of mental disorders III (1980 3rd ed. DSM-III) Washington, DC

American Psychiatric Association: Diagnostic and statistical manual of mental disorders IV (1994 4th ed. DSM-IV) Washington, DC

American Psychiatric Association: Justification of Criteria - Somatic Symptoms DRAFT 4/18/11. 2011; Washington, DC

American Psychiatric Association: Diagnostic and statistical manual of mental disorders III (2013 5th ed. DSM-5) Washington, DC

American Psychiatric Association 2018 https://www.appi.org/permissions & https://webapps.psychiatry.org/RequestForm/

Creed F, Barsky A: A systematic review of the epidemiology of somatisation disorder and hypochondriasis. J Psychosom Res 2004; 56:391-408

Creed F: Can DSM-V facilitate productive research into the somatoform disorders? J Psychosom Res 2006; 60:331–4.

Davis LJ: The Encyclopedia of Insanity. Harper's Magazine 1997; 2:61-6

De Gucht V, Maes S. Explaining medically unexplained symptoms: toward a multidimensional, theory-based approach to somatization. J Psychosom Res 2006; 60:349–52

Dimsdale J, Sharma N, Sharp M: What do physicians think of somatoform disorders? Psychosomatics 2011; 52:154-9

Dimsdale JE, Creed F, Escobar J, Sharpe M, Wulsin L, Barsky A, Lee S, Irwin MR, Levenson J: Somatic symptom disorder: an important change in DSM. J Psychosom Res 2013; 75:223-8

Dirckx JH: Hybrid words in medical terminology. JAMA 1977; 238:2043-5

Fink P, Rosendal M, Olesen F: Classification of somatization and functional somatic symptoms in primary care. Aust NZ J Psychiatry 2005; 39:772–81

Frances AJ: Is DSM 5 A Public Trust Or An APA Cash Cow? Psychology Today 2012, Jan 3 https://www.psychologytoday.com/ca/blog/dsm5-in-distress/201201/is-dsm-5-public-trust-or-apa-cash-cow

Frances AJ: The new somatic symptom disorder in DSM-5 risks mislabeling many people as mentally ill. BMJ 2013; 346:f1580

Gureje O, Reed GM: Bodily distress disorder in ICD-11: problems and prospects. World Psychiatry 2016; 15: 291–2

Hiller W: Don't change a winning horse. J Psychosom Res 2006; 60:345–7

Kroenke K: Physical symptom disorder: a simpler diagnostic category for somatization-spectrum conditions. J Psychosom Res 2006; 60:335–9

Levenson JL: A rose by any other name is still a rose. J Psychosom Res 2006; 60:325–6

Levenson JL: The somatoform disorders: 6 characters in search of an author. Psychiatr Clin North Am 2011; 34:515–24

Lipowski ZJ: Somatization: The concept and its clinical application. Am J Psychiatry 1988; 145:1358-68

Lynch DJ, McGrady A, Nagel R, Zsembik C: Somatization in Family Practice: Comparing 5 Methods of Classification. Primary Care Companion to The Journal of Clinical Psychiatry 1999; 1:85-9

Mai FM, Merskey H: Briquet's Treatise on hysteria. A synopsis and commentary. Arch Gen Psychiatry 1980; 37:1401-5

Mayou R, Kirmayer LJ, Simon G, Kroenke K, Sharpe M: Somatoform disorders: time for a new approach in DSM-V. Am J Psychiatry 2005; 162:847–55

Perley MJ, Guze SB: Hysteria: The stability and usefulness of clinical criteria. New England Journal of Medicine 1962; 266:421-6

Rief W, Sharpe M: Somatoform disorders: new approaches to classification, conceptualization, and treatment. J Psychosom Res 2004; 56:387–90

Robins E, Guze SB: Establishment of diagnostic validity in psychiatric illness: Its application to Schizophrenia. Am J Psychiatry 1970; 126:107-11

Scamvougeras A, Berzen L, Tham J, Howard A, Ilcewicz M, Dimov M, Stowe R, Hurwitz T: Somatoform Disorders; Somatic Symptom Disorders; Intended DSM-5 Changes. (unpublished letter to Members of the DSM-5 Somatic Symptom Disorders Work Group, June 28 2011), see Appendix VI (pp. 195-202)

Sharpe M, Mayou R, Bass C, editors: Treatment of functional somatic symptoms. Oxford. Oxford University Press, 1995. p466

Sharpe M, Carson A: "Unexplained" somatic symptoms, functional syndromes, and somatization: do we need a paradigm shift? Ann Intern Med 2001; 134:926–30

Stone J, Smyth R, Carson A, Lewis S, Prescott R, Warlow C, Sharpe M: The misdiagnosis of conversion symptoms/hysteria – a systematic review. BMJ 2005; 331: 989-91

Stone J: Neurologic approaches to hysteria, psychogenic and functional disorders from the late 19th century onwards. In: Functional Neurologic Disorders, Handbook of Clinical Neurology 2016; 139:25-36

Trimble M, Reynolds EH: A brief history of hysteria: From the ancient to the modern. In: Functional Neurologic Disorders, Handbook of Clinical Neurology 2016; 139:3-10

World Health Organization: The ICD-10 classification of mental and behavioural disorders: clinical descriptions and diagnostic guidelines. WHO 1992. Geneva.

World Health Organization. ICD-11 Beta Draft: 6C60 Bodily Distress Disorder. 2018 Available at https://icd.who.int/dev11/l-m/en#/http://id.who.int/icd/entity/767044268

Ziegler DK, Paul N: On the natural history of hysteria in women. Diseases of the Nervous System 1954; 15:3–8

APPENDIX II

RISK OF MISDIAGNOSIS

The Risk of Misdiagnosis in Somatoform Disorders

Handling diagnostic uncertainty is one of the many challenges in the accurate assessment and management of complicated patients with Somatoform Disorders. Some authors have published rates of misdiagnosis as primary outcomes where others have reported diagnostic changes as part of follow-up studies. Despite the heterogeneity in the reports, over thirty articles can be found in the literature illustrating the possible causes and rates of misdiagnosis, and some conclusions can be drawn from that body of information. Clinicians working with somatoform patients can be somewhat reassured that studies have consistently disclosed lower than 15% misdiagnosis rates (Mace & Trimble 1996, Moene 2000) for the last forty years or more. Prior to that, as many as 30% of some patient groups were later found to have non-psychiatric conditions that may have explained patients' presenting symptoms (Slater 1965a). This decrease in clinician error precedes the advent of sophisticated ancillary neuropsychiatric diagnostic techniques, such as neuroimaging. It likely reflects a change in the methodology of studies in this area or a change in the accuracy of clinicians' assessments and re-assessments.

Several reports in recent years show a negligible risk of misdiagnosis (4% or less) but those are often from tertiary care centres with referral and sampling biases, in patients with longer duration of illness or shorter follow-up periods, with non-psychiatric (especially neurological) comorbidity excluded (Couprie 1995, Crimlisk 1996, Binzer 1998). There is little question that misdiagnosis still occurs. A central issue is whether the misdiagnosis rate in Somatoform Disorders at this point in time is higher than for other neurological or psychiatric conditions. One of the most comprehensive reviews on this subject looked at previously reported studies between 1965 and 2003 that included at least 10 patients over the age of 16 with somatoform symptoms of duration greater than 6 months (Stone 2005). The authors reported a misdiagnosis rate of 8.4% (123 of 1466 cases with adequate follow-up). There were also up to 30 additional cases diagnosed with psychogenic amplification of neurological symptoms that were likely also misdiagnosed. There was a median follow-up rate in the studies of 86% and median follow-up time of 5 years. The review excluded studies with patients with Somatoform Pain Disorder and Somatization Disorder although these conditions are generally met with less diagnostic uncertainty than some of the pseudoneurological syndromes such as nonepileptic seizures or psychogenic movement disorders.

The literature in this area is limited by retrospective data with few studies comprehensively re-evaluating patients on follow-up (most studies rely on telephone interviews with patients and/or family physicians' notes). Exclusion criteria and patient selection vary considerably. Methods of reporting and assessing symptoms are heterogeneous. Despite these differences, which likely account for the substantial inconsistency in misdiagnosis rates, there is much to be learned about diagnostic pitfalls. Clinician error not uncommonly results from: bizarre symptomatology; the presence of a psychiatric history; a preceding psychologically traumatic event; an absence of physical findings or the presence of atypical findings on examination; a lack of concern on behalf of the patient ("la belle indifference"); an improvement seen with suggestion or narcoanalysis; decisions based on duration of symptoms, severity of dysfunction, or multitude of complaints; and abnormal illness behaviour including over-dramatization (Lang 2006). This preceding list generally contains helpful diagnostic clues for the clinician but the point of the literature is that any one diagnostic clue in the absence of others may represent a "fertile source of clinical error," as Slater (1965b) cautiously put it. Despite these cautions, the medical literature would support the approach of a thorough assessment, and communication with the patient about the low probability of misdiagnosis. It also supports the need for careful ongoing monitoring for the possible emergence of signs of a general medical condtion, perhaps with regular re-examination by a non-psychiatric specialist. A measured diagnosis of Somatoform Disorder, appreciative of the possibility of error, will avoid harm from inappropriate investigations, and will eliminate the delay in properly initiating management in these patients, a delay which could worsen their prognosis and cause undue physical harm through the chronicity of the condition and all the consequences of the person remaining ill.

References:

Binzer M, Kullgren G: Motor Conversion Disorder: A Prospective 2- to 5-Year Follow-Up Study. Psychosomatics 1998; 39:519-27

Couprie W, Wijdicks EFM, Rooijmans HGM, van Gijn J: Outcome in conversion disorder: a follow up study. J Neurol Neurosurg Psychiatry 1995; 58:750-2

Crimlisk HL, Bhatia K, Cope H, David A, Marsden CD, Ron MA: Slater revisited: 6 year follow-up study of medically unexplained motor symptoms. BMJ 1998; 316:582-6

Lang, AE: General Overview of Psychogenic Movement Disorders: Epidemiology, Diagnosis, and Prognosis. In: Hallett M, Fahn S, Jankovik J, Lang AE, Cloninger CR, Yudofsky SC eds. Psychogenic Movement Disorders. Lippincott, Williams & Wilkins: Philadelphia, 2006.

Mace CJ, Trimble MR: Ten-Year Prognosis of Conversion Disorder. Br J of Psychiatry 1996; 169:282-8

Moene FC, Landberg EH, Hoogduin KAL, Spinhoven P, Herzberger LI, Kleyweg RP, Weeda J: Organic syndromes diagnosed as conversion disorder: identification and frequency in a study of 85 patients. Journal of Psychosomatic Research 2000; 49:7-12

Slater ETO, Glithero E: A Follow-Up of Patients Diagnosed as Suffering from "Hysteria." Journal of Psychosomatic Research 1965a; 9:9-13.

Slater E: Diagnosis of "Hysteria." BMJ 1965b; 1:1395-9

Stone J, Smyth R, Carson A, Lewis S, Prescott R, Warlow C, Sharpe M: The misdiagnosis of conversion symptoms/hysteria – a systematic review. BMJ 2005; 331: 989-91.

APPENDIX III

PATHOPHYSIOLOGY - A REVIEW

The Pathophysiology of Somatoform Disorders: A Literature Review

It has long been recognized that somatization may occur in the course of organic brain syndromes or may be preceded by a physical trauma or incident (Whitlock 1967). This has prompted a search for more than psychological explanations of the process. Over the last few decades, empirical research into the pathophysiology and neurobiology of somatoform disorders has led us to some intriguing insights. Firstly, the conceptualizations of early practitioners in this field bear some resemblance to our evolving understanding of this clinical problem. Secondly, there is growing evidence of the neurophysiological associations, if not organic etiologies, of the symptoms and psychological underpinnings of conditions characterized by somatization. Lastly, dysfunction in specific circuits in the brain appears to correlate with disease states and may be measurable.

Kozlowska (2005, 2007) and Hallett et al. (2016) provide excellent reviews of historical models of conversion disorder, in conjunction with a presentation of current models. We are reminded that early descriptions of motor symptoms in patients with "hysteria" were compared to the instinctual self-preservation behaviours in animals. The incentives for freezing and appeasement behaviour, often manifested by limb immobility and other pseudoneurological symptoms in toddlers and preschool age children, appear to be: a) self-protection when threatened, and b) stabilization of interpersonal attachments through affective inhibition and distress signalling (Kozlowska 2007). Pioneers in the study of "hysteria" such as Briquet and Charcot also speculated that, in susceptible individuals, a global brain disturbance, or stress and environmental situations, could also disturb the "affective" areas in the nervous system, thus producing symptoms. Our current understanding of the underlying biological mechanisms of conversion disorder is bringing together these seemingly disparate speculations. Recent data suggests that incorrect information may be introduced into patients' representations of their body states or these representations may be omitted from consciousness, allowing for unconscious motor programs associated with innate or learned emotional responses to manifest.

In the past, evidence of a biological pathophysiological basis in somatization was unclear although studies in hysterical anaesthesia demonstrated that evoked potentials of the affected limb had smaller amplitudes than the unaffected side, suggesting some form of corticofugal inhibition (perhaps of the reticular formation) impairing attention to the incoming signal (Whitlock 1967). The source of the patients' pathological attention to physical symptoms is still a major area of inquiry with neurophysiological evidence that sensory signals may not be appropriately filtered (Witthoft 2010). Genetic studies indicating the familial clustering of somatization with antisocial personality disorder and alcohol dependence have appeared to point to some heritability (Mai 2004). Functional symptoms demonstrate modest genetic influences (Henningsen & Creed 2010). Animal models highlight the significance of early life stress in promoting hyperalgesia through presumed alterations in nociceptor signaling (Alvarez 2013, Green 2011).

Other preliminary observations from case reports and case series have helped to define the neurophysiology of Somatoform Disorders. Neurochemical changes in monoaminergic systems occur in somatoform patients even in the absence of overt depression (Reif 2004). Changes in somatosensory evoked potentials (Yazicki 2004) and on SPECT imaging (Tiihonen 1995, Vuilleumier 2001) in affected patients resolve with recovery of the illness. Somatoform Disorders appear to be more common after a brain lesion especially involving the basal ganglia and thalamus (Eames 1992) and a morphometric MRI study suggested women with conversion disorder demonstrated significantly smaller left and right basal ganglia and thalami compared to healthy controls (Atmaca 2006). Functional imaging studies (fMRI, PET) in patients with hysterical anaesthesia (Mailis-Gagnon 2003, Ghaffar 2006), paralysis (Marshall 1997, de Lange 2007) and hypnotically induced paralysis (Halligan 2000), medically unexplained visual loss (Werring 2004), pain amplification (Dimsdale & Dantzer 2007), psychogenic movement disorders (Voon 2010a), and more specifically, psychogenic tremor (Voon 2011), indicate dysfunction in the rostral cingulate as well as aberrant function of the amygdala and connectivity of the cingulate and amygdala with sensorimotor and heteromodal cortical areas. Aberrant amygdala activity in Somatoform Disorders, dissociated from depression and anxiety, may reflect a heightened state of arousal or a failure of attentional processes to adapt to detect threat (Voon 2010b). Increased cingulate activity, with or without involvement of the orbitofrontal cortex, may be a reflection of excessive inhibition, disordered attention to sensorimotor processes, or altered self-monitoring (Hurwitz & Prichard 2006, Van Beilen 2010, Voon 2013). The aberrant functioning of the default mode network, typically decreased during goal-directed tasks and responsible for heightened self-monitoring and the contribution of internal processes to motor function, is a recurrent finding in motor functional neurologic disorders (Voon 2016).

Numerous physical findings, seen with EMG and other techniques, have been measured in patients with so-called "functional somatic syndromes" (Sharpe & Bass 1992, Hallett 2016). Psychogenic movement disorders, including functional tremor, myoclonus, and dystonia, display characteristic features in electrophysiological and neuroimaging studies (Kamble & Pal 2016, Czarnecki 2011). Patients with psychogenic nonepileptic seizures (PNES) are twice as likely to demonstrate abnormal interictal epileptiform discharges on EEG compared to healthy controls (Reuber 2002). Resting EEGs in these patients also show a variety of weakened neural connections, in particular decreased prefrontal and parietal synchronization, which could imply deficient feedforward signaling mechanisms (Knyazeva 2011; Barzegaran 2012 & 2016). Resting fMRI and FDG-PET studies give further evidence in this population of abnormalities in the connectivity and/or functioning of multiple regions including the inferior parietal and anterior cingulate cortices (Arthuis 2014), supramarginal gyrus, insula, precentral sulcus, and intraparietal sulcus (van der Kruijs 2014). Functional imaging has also repeatedly dissociated conversion paralysis from feigned weakness (Spence 2000, Stone 2007, Cojan 2009) and has speculated on alternative deficits to motor inhibition in conversion paralysis such as failure to initiate motor activity or a failure to conceptualize movement (Burgmer 2006). Associations between the degree of somatization and fluctuations in cortisol levels (Rief 1998), systolic blood pressure (Kristal-Boneh

1998), reduced cytokine-mediated immune function (Gil 2007), and other markers of physiological arousal (galvanic skin response, startle response, reduced heart rate variability) (Tak & Rosmalen 2009, Maurer 2016) including impaired amygdala habituation (Voon 2010b, Aybek 2015) have been seen, regardless of psychopathological distress. There are models suggesting limited prefrontal control of the sympathetic and parasympathetic nervous systems, citing particular evidence that reduced parasympathetic activity is found generally amongst a multitude of functional somatic syndromes (Henningsen & Creed 2010). Whether these findings are causal in the clinical disturbance has yet to be determined.

Recent investigations have attempted to uncover how the facilitation or inhibition of a movement might be perceived as involuntary despite the involvement of voluntary mechanisms. Edwards et al. (2012) propose that specific motor or sensory outcomes are afforded undue attention, perhaps as a result of a physical precipitant such as injury or infection. The patient then develops incorrect beliefs regarding illness-related sensations or movements, and these become the subject of aberrant attentional bias. The top-down "priors" override bottom-up stimulus information but do not predict the content of the precepts themselves, thus contributing to a sense of loss of agency over one's symptoms. Perez et al. (2012) present a functional unawareness theory in unilateral motor and somatosensory functional neurological disorders (FNDs), similar to patients who suffer from right-sided lesions and resultant hemispheric neglect. This is supported by previous evidence that dysfunction of right hemisphere structures tends to result more frequently in conversion symptoms than when dysfunction occurs in the left hemisphere. For example, right anterior temporal lobectomies in seizure patients more commonly precipitate conversion disorder, regardless of the patient's handedness (Devinsky 2001). Parees et al. (2014) propose that decreased sensory attenuation for self-generated movements underlies the perception of involuntariness in functional movement disorders. Regarding specific pathways involved in patients' loss of self-agency, disconnection of the supplementary motor area and other cortical regions is thought to result in disinhibition of unwanted actions, which allows previously mapped conversion motor representations to be activated in an unchecked fashion. The concomitant movement is thought to arise without normal prediction of its sensory consequences (Hallett 2016).

A variety of theories have been proposed to unify the neurobiological and imaging findings in the current literature. In simplified terms, the functioning of the primary motor and sensory cortices appear to be generally normal in somatoform disorders, but with notable aberrancies of the premotor cortex, association cortices, and limbic regions. This suggests that top-down dysfunction likely plays a key role in the pathology of pseudoneurological symptoms, with abnormalities of the temporoparietal junction and other areas potentially influencing patients' sense of control over their symptoms (Hallett 2016). Alterations in areas responsible for emotional regulation, which in turn modulates those regions involved in planning as well as execution and attribution of movement, is another potential broad explanation for the pathogenesis of somatization disorder (Lehn 2016).

Perez et al (2015a, 2015b) summarize FNDs as arising from aberrancies of multiple neurological networks including those involved in visceral-somatic perception, emotional processing/regulation/awareness, intentional behaviour, volition, cognitive control, self-referential processing, and motor planning. These pathways include the amygdala, insula, anterior cingulate cortex, dorsolateral prefrontal cortex, supramarginal gyrus, temporoparietal junction, and supplementary motor cortex, which all play specific and interconnected roles in the pathophysiology of these conditions (Voon 2016).

Boeckle et al (2016) propose similar theories in their recent meta-analysis. Disruptions in cortical inhibition (as evidenced by increased primary somatosensory and motor cortex activity of the affected side), voluntary-intentional capacities (due to malfunction of prefrontal areas), attention (increased anterior cingulate cortex, parietal cortex, and striatum activity, plus decreased activity of the thalamus and supramarginal gyrus), action authorship and agency (temporoparietal junction, somatosensory cortex, anterior cingulate cortex, parietal associative cortex, gyrus temporalis superior), affect (amygdala, anterior cingulate cortex), and cortical thickness (premotor cortex, primary motor cortex, cerebellum), are all strongly associated with FNDs.

As the study of the pathophysiology of somatoform conditions continues, the connections between historical and contemporary understanding, and between psychological and physiological explanations of the illness, will no doubt be made. In the meanwhile, these presumed connections could be taken to the bedside to reassure both physicians and patients that an even better understanding awaits us (Sharpe & Bass 1992).

References:

Alvarez P, Green PG, Levine JD: Stress in the adult rat exacerbates muscle pain induced by early-life stress. Biol Psychiatry 2013; 74:688-95

Arthuis M, Micoulaud-Franchi JA, Bartolomei F, McGonigal A, Guedj E: Resting cortical PET metabolic changes in psychogenic non-epileptic seizures (PNES). J Neurol Neurosurg Psychiatry 2015; 86:1106-12

Asadi-Pooya AA: Biological underpinnings of psychogenic nonepileptic seizures: directions for future research. Neurol Sci 2016; 37:1033-8

Atmaca M, Aydin A, Tezcan E, Poyraz AK, Kara B: Volumetric investigation of brain regions in patients with conversion disorder. Progress in Neuro-Psychopharmacology & Biological Psychiatry 2006; 30:708-13

Aybek S, Nicholson TR, O'Daly O, Zelaya F, Kanaan RA, David AS: Emotion-motion interactions in conversion disorder: an fMRI study. PLoS One 2015; 10(4):e0123273

Barzegaran E, Carmeli C, Rossetti AO, Frackowiak RS, Knyazeva MG: Weakened functional connectivity in patients with psychogenic non-epileptic seizures (PNES) converges on basal ganglia. J Neurol Neurosurg Psychiatry 2016; 87:332-7

Barzegaran E, Joudaki A, Jalili M, Rossetti AO, Frackowiak RS, Knyazeva MG: Properties of functional brain networks correlate with frequency of psychogenic non-epileptic seizure. Front Hum Neurosci 2012; 6:335

Boeckle M, Liegl G, Jank R, Pieh C: Neural correlates of conversion disorder: overview and meta-analysis of neuroimaging studies on motor conversion disorder. BMC Psychiatry 2016; 16:195

Burgmer , Konrad C, Jansen A, Kugel H, Sommer J, Heindel W, Ringelstein EB, Heuft G, Knecht S: Abnormal brain activation during movement observation in patients with conversion paralysis. NeuroImage 2006; 29:1336-43

Cojan Y, Waber L, Carruzzo A, Vuilleumier P: Motor inhibition in hysterical conversion paralysis. Neuroimage 2009; 47:1026-37

Czarnecki K, Jones DT, Burnett MS, Mullan B, Matsumoto JY: SPECT perfusion patterns distinguish psychogenic from essential tremor. Parkinsonism Relat Disord 2011; 17:328-32

de Lange FP, Roelofs K, Toni I: Increased self-monitoring during imagined movements in conversion paralysis. Neuropsychologia 2007; 45:2051-8

de Lange FP, Toni I, Roelofs K: Altered connectivity between prefrontal and sensorimotor cortex in conversion paralysis. Neuropsychologia 2010; 48: 1782-8

Devinsky O, Mesad S, Alper K: Nondominant Hemisphere Lesions and Conversion Nonepileptic Seizures. Journal of Neuropsychiatry and Clinical Neurosciences 2001; 13: 367-73

Dimsdale JE, Dantzer R: A Biological Substrate for Somatoform Disorders: Importance of Pathophysiology. Psychosomatic Medicine 2007; 69:850-4

Eames P: Hysteria following brain injury. J Neurol Neurosurg Psychiatry 1992; 55:1046-53

Edwards MJ, Adams RA, Brown H, Parees I, Friston KJ: A Bayesian account of 'hysteria'. Brain 2012; 135:3495-512

Ghaffar O, Staines WR, & A Feinstein: Unexplained neurologic symptoms: an fMRI study of sensory conversion disorder. Neurology 2006; 67:2036-8

Gil FP, Nickel M, Ridout N, Schwarz M, Schoechlin C, Schmidmaier R: Alexithymia and Interleukin Variations in Somatoform Disorder. Neuroimmunomodulation 2007; 14:235-42

Green PG, Chen X, Alvarez P, Ferrari LF, Levine JD: Early-life stress produces muscle hyperalgesia and nociceptor sensitization in the adult rat. Pain 2011; 152:2549-556

Halligan PW, Athwal BS, Oakley DA, Frackowiak RSJ: Imaging hypnotic paralysis: implications for conversion hysteria. Lancet 2000; 355:986-7

Hallett M. Physiology of psychogenic movement disorders. Journal of Clinical Neuroscience 2010; 17:959-65

Hallett M, Stone J, Carson A: *Handbook of Clinical Neurology* 2016; Vol.139. Academic Press.

Henningsen P, Creed F: The genetic, physiological, and psychological mechanisms underlying disabling medically unexplained symptoms and somatisation. Journal of Psychosomatic Research 2010; 68:395-7

Hurwitz TA, Prichard JW: Conversion disorder and fMRI. Neurology 2006; 67:1914-5

Kamble NL, Pal PK: Electrophysiological evaluation of psychogenic movement disorders. Parkinsonism and Related Disorders 2016; 22:S153-8

Kozlowska K: Healing the Disembodied Mind: Contemporary Models of Conversion Disorder. Harvard Review of Psychiatry 2005; 13:1-13K

Kozlowska, K: The Developmental Origins of Conversion Disorders. Clinical Child Psychology and Psychiatry 2007; 12:487-510

Knyazeva MG, Jalili M, Frackowiak RS, Rossetti AO: Psychogenic seizures and frontal disconnection: EEG synchronisation study. J Neurol Neurosurg Psychiatry 2011; 82:505-11

Kristal-Boneh E, Melamed S, Kushnir T, Froom P, Harari G, Ribak J: Association between somatic symptoms and 24-hour ambulatory blood pressure levels. Psychosomatic medicine 1998; 60:616-9

Lehn A, Gelauff J, Hoeritzauer I, Ludwig L, McWhirter L, Williams S, Gardiner P, Carson A, Stone J: Functional neurological disorders: mechanisms and treatment. J Neurol 2016; 263:611-20

Lorenz J, Kunze K, Bromm R: Differentiation of conversive sensory loss and malingering by P300. NeuroReport 1998; 9:187-91

Mai F: Somatization Disorder: A Practical Review. Can J Psychiatry 2004; 49:652-62

Mailis-Gagnon A, Giannoylis I, Downar J, Kwan CL, Mikulis DJ, Crawley AP, Nicholson K, Davis KD: Altered central somatosensory processing in chronic pain patients with hysterical anesthesia. Neurology 2003; 60:1501-7

Marshall JC, Halligan PW, Fink GR, Wade DT, Frackowiak RS: The functional anatomy of a hysterical paralysis. Cognition 1997; 64:B1-8

Maurer CW, Liu VD, LaFaver K, Ameli R, Wu T, Toledo R, Epstein SA, Hallett M: Impaired resting vagal tone in patients with functional movement disorders. Parkinsonism Relat Disord 2016; 30:18-22

Naga AA, Devinsky O, Barr WB: Somatoform Disorders After Temporal Lobectomy. Cog Behav Neurol 2004; 17:57-61

Parees I, Brown H, Nuruki A, Adams RA, Davare M, Bhatia KP, Friston K, Edwards MJ: Loss of sensory attenuation in patients with functional (psychogenic) movement disorders. Brain 2014; 137:2916-21

Perez DL, Barsky AJ, Daffner K, Silbersweig DA: Motor and somatosensory conversion disorder: a functional unawareness syndrome? J Neuropsychiatry Clin Neurosci 2012; 24:141-51

Perez DL, Barsky AJ, Vago DR, Baslet G, Silbersweig DA: A neural circuit framework for somatosensory amplification in somatoform disorders. J Neuropsychiatry Clin Neurosci 2015a; 27:40-50

Perez DL, Dworetazky BA, Dickerson BC, Leung L, Cohn R, Baslet G, Silbersweig DA: An integrative neurocircuit perspective on psychogenic nonepileptic seizures and functional movement disorders: neural functional unawareness. Clin EEG Neurosci 2015b; 46:4-15

Reuber M, Fernandez G, Bauer J, Singh DD, Elger CE: Interictal EEG abnormalities in patients with psychogenic nonepileptic seizures. Epilepsia 2002; 43:1013-20

Rief W, Shaw R, Fichter MM: Elevated levels of psychophysiological arousal and cortisol in patients with somatization syndrome. Psychosomatic medicine 1998; 60:198-203

Rief, Pilger F, Ihle D, Verkerk R, Scharpe S, Maes M: Psychobiological Aspects of Somatoform Disorders: Contributions of Monoaminergic Transmitter Systems. Neuropsychobiology 2004; 49: 24-9

Sharpe M, Bass C: Pathophysiological Mechanisms in Somatization. Int Rev Psychiatry 1992; 40:81-97

Spence SA, Crimlisk HL, Cope H, Ron MA, Grasby PM: Discrete neurophysiological correlates in prefrontal cortex during hysterical and feigned disorder of movement. Lancet 2000; 355:1243-4

Stone J, Zeman A, Simonottoa E, Meyer M, Azuma R, Flett S, Sharpe M: fMRI in Patients With Motor Conversion Symptoms and Controls With Simulated Weakness. Psychosomatic Medicine 2007; 69:961-9

Tak LM, Rosmalen JGM: Dysfunction of stress responsive systems as a risk factor for functional somatic syndromes. Journal of Psychosomatic Research 2009; 68:461-8

Tiihonen J, Kuikka J, Viinamaki H, Lehtonen J, Partanen J: Altered cerebral blood flow during hysterical paresthesia. Biological Psychiatry 1995; 37:134-5

Van Beilen M, Vogt BA, Leenders KL: Increased activation in cingulate cortex in conversion disorder: What does it mean? Journal of the Neurological Sciences 2010; 289:155-8

van der Kruijs SJ, Jagannathan SR, Bodde NM, Besseling RM, Lazeron RH, Vonck KE, Boon PA, Cluitmans PJ, Hofman PA, Backes WH, Aldenkamp AP, Jansen JF: Resting-state networks and dissociation in psychogenic non-epileptic seizures. J Psychiatr Res 2014; 54:126-33

Voon V, Gallea C, Hattori N, Bruno M, Ekanayake V, Hallett M: The involuntary nature of conversion disorder. Neurology 2010a; 74:223-8

Voon V, Brezing C, Gallea C, Ameli R, Roelofs K, Curt LaFrance Jr W, Hallett M: Emotional stimuli and motor conversion disorder. Brain 2010b; 133:1526-36

Voon V, Brezing C, Gallea C, Hallet M: Aberrant supplementary motor complex and limbic activity during motor preparation in motor conversion disorder. Mov Disord 2011; 26:2396-2403

Voon V, Ekanayake V, Wiggs E, Kranick S, Ameli R, Harrison NA, Hallett M: Response inhibition in motor conversion disorder. Mov Disord 2013; 28:612-8

Voon V, Cavanna AE, Cobum K, Sampson S, Reeve A, LaFrance WC: Functional neuroanatomy and neurophysiology of functional neurological disorders (conversion disorder). J Neuropsychiatry Clin Neurosci 2016; 28:168-190

Vuilleumier P: Functional neuroanatomical correlates of hysterical sensorimotor loss. Brain 2001; 124:1077-90

Vuilleumier P: Hysterical conversion and brain function. Progress in Brain Research 2005; 150:309-29

Werring DJ, Weston L, Bullmore ET, Plant GT, Ron MA: Functional magnetic resonance imaging of the cerebral response to visual stimulation in medically unexplained visual loss. Psychological Medicine 2004; 34:583-9

Whitlock, FA: The Aetiology of Hysteria. Acta Psychiatrica Scandinavica 1967; 43:144-62

Witthoft M, Hiller W: Psychological Approaches to Origins and Treatments of Somatoform Disorders. Annual Review of Clinical Psychology 2010; 6:257-83

Yazici KM, Demirci M, Demir B, Ertugrul A: Abnormal SSEPs in two patients with conversion disorder. Psychiatry and Clinical Neurosciences 2004; 58:222-5

Yazici KM, Kostakoglu L: Cerebral blood flow changes in patients with conversion disorder. Psychiatry Research 1998; 83:163-8

APPENDIX IV

MANAGEMENT - A REVIEW

The Management of Somatoform Disorders: A Literature Review

The literature on somatization focuses more on the prevalence, classification, diagnosis, and cost to patients and society than on the management of this complex problem (Janca 2006). Observations on treatment are fraught with methodological difficulties. There is a limited generalizability of most samples analyzed due to the complicated heterogeneity of patients with somatization, and studies often lack a control group or adequate follow-up, making the exact agent of change difficult to determine (Mai 2004). Intention-to-treat analyses and randomization are rarely utilized and few studies are long-term in a population prone to relapse (Allen 2002). It often proves difficult to dissociate physical and psychiatric outcomes, and evaluations are often performed by unblinded clinicians (Lidbeck 2003). Pharmacological and psychological interventions have not been compared (Sumathipala 2007). Patients with multiple functional somatic syndromes, but lacking a formal psychiatric diagnosis, have not been thoroughly studied, while there is extensive research on singular specific functional syndromes (e.g. irritable bowel syndrome, fibromyalgia, and chronic fatigue syndrome, amongst others), which often recommends interventions that are also helpful in patients with DSM-IV somatoform disorders (Henningsen 2007). The newer DSM-5 classification of Somatic Symptom Disorders also alters the patient population that falls under the broad category of somatoform conditons, by necessitating positive psychological symptoms and removing the requirement of symptoms being medically unexplained (Rief & Martin 2014, Van Dessel 2016). Despite the complications of examining this population, there are a number of studies outlining both the general principles of management and specific interventions to be considered.

For practitioners managing patients with somatoform conditions in primary care, a number of principles may apply. One should take time to educate the patient and the family, explain what the illness is and is not and how the diagnosis was determined, encourage patients to re-attribute symptoms to likely etiologies, and make attempts to reassure the patient that no underlying non-psychiatric conditions have been missed, often by providing regular scheduled visits with brief physical examinations (Mai 2004, Stone 2005, Janca 2006, Stone & Sharpe 2006). Psychiatric consultation is strongly encouraged, and has been shown to improve physical functioning and decrease health care costs after 2 years (Smith 1995, Kroenke 2007). Effective communication to the mental health professional that the physical symptoms are in fact atypical according to non-psychiatric specialists will avoid doubt of the diagnosis by consultants and by the patient (Hinson & Haren 2006).

Each intensive approach to the patient with somatization should begin with a comprehensive assessment of the medical, psychiatric, and psychosocial aspects of the case (Lipowski 1988). The diagnosis should be made and treatment initiated as early as possible (Lloyd 1989). Communicating to the patient an understanding of the condition and providing information on cause, prevalence, and treatment (as one would do for any other medical problem) may be the most important step in management (Oyama 2007).

Physicians are in the optimal position to explain the results of the neurological and general physical exam signs that delineate between functional and psychological symptoms to reassure patients of a non-organic cause to their symptoms (Daum 2014, Tsui 2017). There should be reassurance that the etiology is not sinister albeit distressing, the pathophysiological mechanism is involuntary, and the illness is real not "faked" (Stone 2005, Chaturvedi 2006, Ali 2015). The patient's distress should be validated and it should be emphasized that, in medicine, the degree of suffering often does not correlate with the extent of tissue damage (Servan-Schreiber 2000). The explanation should be empowering, involving a link between physiological and psychological factors, and should neither collude with the patient's misattributions nor reject symptoms as "all in one's head" (Salmon 1999). The terms 'functional' and 'non-organic' are favoured by the patient over 'psychogenic,' when providing a diagnosis to a patient (Ding & Kanaan 2017).

Examples of other more socially acceptable stress-related diseases, such as stress-related hypertension, can help normalize the symptoms for the patient (Ali 2015). Authors vary in their support for "pseudoscientific" explanations (Speed 1996), physiological or neurological explanations (Kirmayer 2004, Stone & Sharpe 2006), and reference to the role of the brain (Silver 1996). It is proposed that the formulation should be honest, resting on the diagnosis and treatment as psychiatric, and should be accompanied by an unambiguous presentation of findings (Zwillich 1999). Other authors suggest that the focus should be on a common problem in the nervous system that is causing a disturbance in function and that is reversible (Stone & Sharpe 2006). Spurious diagnoses and mind-body dualism should be avoided as it only reinforces hostility and distrust (Lipowski 1988, Bass & Benjamin 1993).

Careful attention to the relationship with the patient is required and may be facilitated by an unbiased exploration of the patients' beliefs and worries about the illness (Mayou 1993, Rosebush & Mazurek 2011). Practitioners should maintain interest in the patient and a focus on functioning rather than symptoms. As the treatment progresses, time between visits can be slowly increased (Murphy 1982). It is encouraged that the treating clinician remains challenging but hopeful (Speed 1996), conveying an expectation of recovery to the patient (Silver 1996). It may be helpful to explore previous responses to physicians (Bass & Benjamin 1993). A common warning is to limit the number of physicians involved as well as unnecessary investigations and treatments, including habit-forming and as needed or "prn" medications, especially opiate analgesics (Mayou 1993, Smith 1995, Servan-Schreiber 2000, Mai 2004). It can be helpful to involve significant others in treatment sessions in order to facilitate understanding, as well as have family reinforce information provided by physicians (Woolfolk 2017, LaFrance 2013). Specific interventions were previously limited to the hope for spontaneous remission, suggestion, hypnosis, narco-analysis (e.g. amytal interviews), environmental manipulation, functional electric stimulation, medications for associated conditions, and EMG biofeedback (Silver 1996). Due to a concern that some patients may have consciously elaborated their symptoms, "strategic" behavioural therapy was applied to inpatients systematically, administering the belief that the persistence of symptoms suggested a psychiatric etiology. However, the ethics of this intervention were questioned and many patients relapsed (Shapiro 2004).

Observations from more recent investigations suggest potential efficacy of other modalities of treatment. Data on pharmacotherapy is limited although the use of antidepressants, both conventional and 'alternative' including St. John's Wort, may be helpful in somatization even in the absence of dysphoria (Okugawa 1992, Menza 2001, Fallon 2004, Kleinstauber 2014). Fluoxetine, escitalopram, and venlafaxine, amongst others have been shown to reduce somatic symptom severity (Kleinstauber 2014). Studies which could systematically dissociate the beneficial effects of antidepressants and antipsychotics in treating symptoms of anxiety and depression, as opposed to somatic symptoms, have not been completed (Kroenke 2007). The use of antidepressants and anticonvulsants in patients with pain has been documented (Janca 2006). Antidepressants have been reported to help patients with psychogenic movement disorders without somatization disorder (Voon & Lang 2005). Haloperidol and more advantageously sulpiride have been examined in conversion disorder (Rampello 1996) and ECT for patients with nonepileptic seizures amongst other conversion disorders may provide benefit (Blumer 2009, Leong 2015). Physical therapy, relaxation training, sleep hygiene, exercise and alleviating the fear that exercise will exacerbate symptoms, involvement of family members in assessment and treatment, and behavioural therapy as an inpatient or outpatient, to unlearn maladaptive behavioural responses to symptoms, and assertive treatment of psychiatric and non-psychiatric co-morbidity have all been recommended (Sharpe & Bass 1992, Speed 1996, Mai 2004, Stone 2005, Rosebush & Mazurek 2011).

Psychosocial treatment, including progressive muscle relaxation, short-term dynamic psychotherapy, hypnotherapy, relaxation, stress management, and EMG biofeedback, have been shown to have a modest impact on disability and physical discomfort, but lasting and clinically meaningful effects have not yet been noted (Allen 2002). Cognitive-behavioural therapy is the most studied model with individual and group administration in somatoform conditions but not in conversion or somatoform pain disorders. In uncertain dosages and at uncertain stages of the patient's illness, it has been shown to be effective even in the chronic and debilitated patients, with gain maintained in less impaired patients up to at least 18 months (Looper & Kirmayer 2002, Bleichhardt 2004, Kroenke 2007, Allen & Woolfolk 2010, Moreno 2013, Van Dessel 2014). While patients may not always rate their psychological distress as improved, they may gain a sense of self-control through improved coping, more realistic symptom attribution, less catastrophizing, and diminished avoidant behaviour (Kroenke & Swindle 2000). They rate their somatization as improved, there is more symptom relief, and less health care utilization (Allen & Woolfolk 2010). The authors' own model (Allen & Woolfolk) of affective cognitive behavioural therapy (CBT) (a multimodal intervention with mindfulness, interpersonal techniques, and cognitive-behavioural therapy, amongst others) for somatization has been demonstrated to be effective in primary care models and in patients with moderate to severe somatization. Therapist guided internet-based CBT has been studied as a potential new avenue for efficiently delivering therapy to patients (Hedman 2016). The effect of more psychodynamically oriented psychotherapies is a matter of debate although most authors believe that enhanced emotional awareness is beneficial for somatizing patients (Abbass 2005, Waller & Scheidt 2006). Psychodynamic therapy, which emphasizes emotion expression and exploration of interpersonal relationships, is suggested to be more effective in improving overall functioning than CBT in one report (Koelen 2014). Mindfulness-based therapies, which incorporate CBT with mindfulness meditation, have also been shown to have a positive effect on the severity of symptoms (Fjorback 2013, Lakhan & Schofield 2013, Van Dessel 2014).

Inpatient treatment has been explored for more complicated patients or for patients in environments that deter their recovery (Rosebush & Mazurek 2011, Saifee 2012). A drug-assisted interview or narco-analysis may benefit patients with acute or treatment-resistant conversion disorder (Poole & Agrawal 2010). An interdisciplinary team in a rehabilitation hospital has been shown to be effective for patients with conversion disorder with motor symptoms (Heruti 2002). Physical rehabilitation for some patients may be highly therapeutic (Stone & Sharpe 2006). A rehabilitation team that focuses specifically on adapted physical activity demonstrated improved physical function in patients with psychogenic gait disorder (Jordbru 2014). To help more persistent somatizers, a multi-axial Psychosomatic Medicine Unit in a psychiatric hospital was established (Abbey & Lipowski 1987). If patients are managed by a team, it is important that effective communication is maintained amongst team members with regards to the unconscious nature of the disturbance and to establish a consensus on the best approach to reinforcing and extinguishing the patients' adaptive and maladaptive behaviours (Speed 1996).

Preventative and health management interventions are also necessary. This should include improved training in and facilities for the assessment and treatment of patients with somatization (Mayou 1993). Efforts should also be made to educate the public and clinicians about the involuntary nature of the illness (Smith 1995) and to further our understanding of the mechanism of somatization, although empirical evidence of clinician education in the absence of collaborative care has not been shown to improve patient outcomes thus far. We are aware of only one paper that attempted to prevent somatization in primary care (Rosendal 2007). A psychoeducation program educating patients about hypochondriasis and the attribution of physical symptoms did not alter the prevalence of somatoform disorders in the sample after five years but did decrease overt psychiatric morbidity, anxiety and depression scores, and perception of general health (Garcia-Campayo 2010). A collaborative care model in an outpatient setting involving training for general practitioners as well as access to psychiatric consultation is beneficial for patients (van der Feltz-Cornelis 2012). Lastly, clinicians at all levels working with this population should be taught how to deal more effectively with the psychological challenges presented by patients with unexplained medical symptoms (Kirmayer 2004).

References:

Abbass A: Somatization: Diagnosing it sooner through emotion-focused interviewing. The Journal of Family Practice 2005; 54:231-243

Abbey SE, Lipowski ZJ. Comprehensive management of persistent somatization: an innovative inpatient program. Psychotherapy and Psychosomatics 1997; 48:110-5

Ali S, Jabeen S, Pate RJ, Shahid M, Chinala S, Nathani M, Shah R: Conversion Disorder - Mind versus Body: A Review. Innov Clin Neurosci 2015; 12:27-33

Allen LA, Escobar JI, Lehrer PM, Gara MA, Woolfolk RL: Psychosocial treatments for multiple unexplained physical symptoms: a review of the literature. Psychosomatic Medicine 2002; 64:939-50

Allen LA, Woolfolk RL: Therapy for Somatoform Disorders. Psychiatr Clin N Am 2010; 33:579-93

Bass C, Benjamin S. The Management of Chronic Somatisation. Brit J Psychiatry 1993; 162:472-80

Bleichhardt G, Timmer B, Rief W: Cognitive-behavioural therapy for patients with multiple somatoform symptoms-a randomized controlled trial in tertiary care. Journal of Psychosomatic Research 2004; 56:449-54

Blumer D, Rice S, Adamolekun B: Electroconvulsive treatment for nonepileptic seizure disorders. Epilepsy & Behavior 2009; 15:382-7

Chaturvedi SK, Desai G, Shaligram D: Somatoform disorders, somatization, and abnormal illness behaviour. International Review of Psychiatry 2006; 18:75-80

Daum C, Hubschmid M, Aybek S: The value of 'positive' clinical signs for weakness, sensory and gait disorders in conversion disorder: a systematic and narrative review. J Neurol Neurosurg Psychiatry 2014; 85:180-90

Ding JM, Kanaan RAA: Conversion disorder: A systematic review of current terminology. General Hospital Psychiatry 2017; 45:51-5

Fallon B: Pharmacotherapy of somatoform disorders. Journal of Psychosomatic Research 2004; 56:455-60

Fjorback LO, Arendt M, Ornbøl E, Walach H, Rehfeld E, Schröder A, Fink P: Mindfulness therapy for somatization disorder and functional somatic syndromes: randomized trial with one-year follow-up. Journal of Psychosomatic Research 2013; 74:31-40

Garcia-Campayo J, Arevalo E, Claraco LM, Alda M, del Hoyo YL: A prevention programme for somatoform disorders is effective for affective disorders. Journal of Affective Disorders 2010; 122:124-32

Hedman E, Axelsson E, Andersson E, Lekander M, Ljótsson B: Exposure-based cognitive-behavioural therapy via the internet and as bibliotherapy for somatic symptom disorder and illness anxiety disorder: randomised controlled trial. Br J Psychiatr 2016; 209:407-13

Henningsen P, Zipfel S, Herzog W: Management of functional somatic syndromes. Lancet 2007; 369: 946-55

Heruti RJ, Levy A, Adunski A, Ohry A: Conversion motor paralysis disorder: overview and rehabilitation model. Spinal Cord 2002; 40:327-34

Hinson VK, Haren WB: Psychogenic Movement Disorders. Lancet Neurol 2006; 5:695-700

Janca A, Isaac M, Ventouras J: Towards better understanding and management of somatoform disorders. International Review of Psychiatry 2006; 18:5-12

Jordbru AA, Smedstad LM, Klungsøyr O, Martinsen EW: Psychogenic gait disorder: a randomized controlled trial of physical rehabilitation with one-year follow-up. J Rehabil Med 2014; 46:181-7

Kirmayer LJ, Groleau D, Looper KJ, Dao MD: Explaining Medically Unexplained Symptoms. Can J Psychiatry 2004; 49:663-72

Kleinstauber M, Witthöft M, Steffanowski A, van Marwijk H, Hiller W, Lambert MJ: Pharmacological interventions for somatoform disorders in adults. Cochrane Database Systematic Reviews 2014; 11:CD010628

Koelen JA, Houtveen JH, Abbass A, Luyten P, Eurelings-Bontekoe EH, Van Broeckhuysen-Kloth SA, Bühring ME, Geenen R: Effectiveness of psychotherapy for severe somatoform disorder: meta-analysis. Br J Psychiatr 2014; 204:12-9

Kroenke K, Swindle R: Cognitive-behavioral therapy for somatization and symptom syndromes: a critical review of controlled clinical trials. Psychother Psychosom 2000; 69:205-15

Kroenke K: Efficacy of Treatment for Somatoform Disorders: A Review of Randomized Controlled Trials. Psychosomatic Medicine 2007; 60:881-8

LaFrance WC, Reuber M, Goldstein LH: Management of psychogenic nonepileptic seizures. Epilepsia 2013; 54:53-67

Lakhan SE, Schofield KL: Mindfulness-based therapies in the treatment of somatization disorders: a systematic review and meta-analysis. PLoS ONE 2013; 8:e71834

Leong KW, Tham JCW, Scamvougeras A, Vila-Rodriguez F: Electroconvulsive therapy treatment in patients with somatic symptom and related disorders. Neuropsychiatric Disease and Treatment 2015; 11:2565-72

Lidbeck J: Group therapy for somatization disorders in primary care: maintenance of treatment goals of short CBT one-and-a-half-year follow-up. Acta Psychiatrica Scandinavica 2003; 107:449-56

Lipowski ZJ: Somatization: the concept and its clinical application. Am J Psychiatry 1988; 145:1358-68

Lloyd G. Somatization: The Psychiatrist's Perspective. Journal of Psychosomatic Research 1989; 33:665-9

Looper KJ, Kirmayer LJ: Behavioral medicine approaches to somatoform disorders. Journal of Consulting and Clinical Psychology 2002; 70:810-27

Mai F. Somatization Disorder: A Practical Review. Can J Psychiatry 2004; 49:652-62

Mayou R: Somatization. Psychotherapy and Psychosomatics 1993; 59:69-83

Menza M, Lauritano M, Allen L, Warman M, Ostella F, Hamer RM, Escobar J: Treatment for somatization disorder with nefazodone: a prospective, open-label study. Ann Clin Psychiatry 2001; 13:153-8

Moreno S, Gili M, Magallón R, Bauzá N, Roca M, Del Hoyo YL, Garcia-Campayo J: Effectiveness of group versus individual cognitive-behavioral therapy in patients with abridged somatization disorder: a randomized controlled trial. Psychosom Med 2013; 75:600-8

Murphy GE: The clinical management of hysteria. JAMA 1982; 247:2559-64

Okugawa G, Yagi A, Kusaka H, Kinoshita T: Paroxetine for Treatment of Somatization Disorder. J Neuropsychiatry Clin Neurosci 2002; 14:464-5

Oyama O, Paltoo C, Greengold J: Somatoform Disorders. Am Fam Phys 2007; 76:1333-8

Poole NA, Agrawal N: Abreaction for conversion disorder: systematic review with meta-analysis. British Journal of Psychiatry 2010; 197:91-5

Rampello I, Raffaele R, Nicoletti G, LePira F, Malaguarnera M, Drago F: Hysterical neurosis of the conversion type: therapeutic activity of neuroleptics with different hyperprolactinemic potency. Neuropsychobiology 1996; 33:186-8

Rief W. Martin A: How to use the new DSM-5 somatic symptom disorder diagnosis in research and practice: a critical evaluation and proposed modifications. Annu Rev Clin Psychol 2014; 10:339-67

Rosebush P, Mazurek M: Treatment of conversion disorder in the 21st century: have we moved beyond the couch? Curr Treat Options Neurol 2011; 13:255-66

Rosendal M, Olesen F, Fink P, Toft T, Sokolowski I, Bro F: A randomized controlled trial of brief training in the assessment and treatment of somatization in primary care: effects on patient outcome. Gen Hosp Psychiatry 2007; 29:364-73

Saifee TA, Kassavetis P, Pareés I, Kojovic M, Fisher L, Morton L, Foong J, Price G, Joyce EM, Edwards MJ: Inpatient treatment of functional motor symptoms: a long-term follow-up study. J Neurol 2012; 259:1958-63

Salmon P, Peters S, Stanley I: Patients' perceptions of medical explanations for somatisation disorders: qualitative analysis. BMP 1999; 318:372-6

Servan-Schreiber D, Tabas G, Kolb NR: Somatizing patients: part II. practical management. Am Fam Physician 2000; 61:1423-8

Shapiro A, Teasell RW: Behavioural interventions in the rehabilitation of acute v. chronic non-organic (conversion/factitious) motor disorders. British Journal of Psychiatry 2004; 185:140-6

Sharpe M, Bass C: Pathophysiological mechanisms in somatization. Int Rev Psychiatry 1992; 40:81-97

Silber TJ: Somatization disorders: diagnosis, treatment, and prognosis. Pediatrics in Review 2011; 32:56-63

Silver FW: Management of conversion disorder. Am J Phys Med Rehab 1996; 75:134-40

Speed J: Behavioural management of conversion disorder: retrospective study. Archives of Physical Medicine and Rehabilitation 1996; 77:147-54

Smith GR, Rost K, Kashner TM: A trial of the effect of a standardized psychiatric consultation on health outcomes and costs in somatizing patients. Archives of General Psychiatry 1995; 52:238-43

Stone J, Carson A, Sharpe M: Functional symptoms in neurology: management. J Neurol Neurosurg Psychiatry 2005; 76:i13-i21

Stone J, Sharpe M: Functional paralysis and sensory disturbance. In Hallett M, Fahn S, Jankovik J, Lang AE, Cloninger CR, Yudofsky SC eds. Psychogenic Movement Disorders. Lippincott Williams & Wilkins: Philadelphia, 2006

Sumathipala A: What is the evidence for the efficacy of treatments for somatoform disorders? A critical review of previous intervention studies. Psychosomatic Medicine 2007; 69:889-900

Tsui P, Deptula A, Yuan DY: Conversion disorder, functional neurological symptom disorder, and chronic pain: comorbidity, assessment, and treatment. Curr Pain Headache Rep 2017; 21:29

van der Fetz-Cornelis CM, Hoedeman R, Keuter EJW, Swinkels JA: Presentation of the multidisciplinary guideline medically unexplained physical symptoms (MUPS) and somatoform disorder in the Netherlands: disease management according to risk profiles. Journal of Psychosomatic Research 2012; 72:168-9

van Dessel N, den Boeft M, van der Wouden JC, Kleinstäuber M, Leone SS, Terluin B, Numans ME, van der Horst HE, van Marwijk H: Non-pharmacological interventions for somatoform disorders and medically unexplained physical symptoms (MUPS) in adults. Cochrane Database Syst Rev 2014; 11:CD011142

van Dessel NC, van der Wouden JC, Dekker J, van der Horst HE: Clinical value of DSM IV and DSM 5 criteria for diagnosing the most prevalent somatoform disorders in patients with medically unexplained physical symptoms (MUPS). J Psychosom Res 2016; 82: 4-10

Voon V, Lang A: Antidepressant outcomes of psychogenic movement disorders. J Clin Psychiatry 2005; 66:1529-34

Waller E, Scheidt CE: Somatoform disorders as disorders of affect regulation: A development perspective. International Review of Psychiatry 2006; 18:13-24

Woolfolk RL, Allen LA, Tiu JE: New directions in the treatment of somatization. Psychiatry Clin N Am 2017; 30: 621-44

Zwillich SH: More thoughts on somatization. Archives of Internal Medicine 1999; 159:1813-4

PATIENT EDUCATION BROCHURE

A Sample Somatoform Disorder Patient Education Brochure

SOMATOFORM DISORDERS

Coping with chronic, disabling, unexplained physical symptoms

What are they?

Thousands of British Columbians have long-term, disabling, unexplained physical symptoms. These symptoms are caused by a process referred to as 'somatization', which occurs when the nervous system, due to significant emotional factors, manifests physical symptoms. The symptoms may last for years despite assessments and recommendations from many doctors.

Symptoms in Somatoform Disorders

Symptoms caused by somatization may include one but more commonly several of the following:

Paralysis
Loss of vision or sensation
Convulsions and spells of altered consciousness
Involuntary movements
Problems with walking
Speech difficulties
Swallowing problems
Pain all over the body or in specific parts such as the arms, legs,

joints, muscles, chest, back, pelvis, genitals, face, and/or jaw; may include headaches
- Gastrointestinal tract dysfunction, such as
  - Nausea with or without vomiting
  - Diarrhea or constipation
  - Bloating
  - Food intolerance
- Fatigue
- Dizziness
- Breathlessness or rapid breathing
- Stronger, faster, or irregular heartbeat
- Difficulty urinating

Clinicians you work with may refer to Somatoform Disorders by various names, including 'Conversion Disorder', 'Bodily Distress Disorders', 'Somatization', 'Somatic Symptom Disorder', 'Functional Neurological Disorder', 'Psychogenic Symptoms'.

How serious are they?

Somatoform Disorders are not life threatening, but they cause much suffering and make it very hard for people to live normal lives. The disorders may be so frustrating that they can even lead to suicidality. The other major risks patients face are side effects or complications from futile and possibly harmful attempts to diagnose and treat their symptoms.

How common are these disorders?

The process of emotional distress occurring physically is universal, with some people experiencing it to a much higher degree than others. At least 35 percent of the population at some point will have physical problems that cause undue duress that remain unexplained despite all appropriate examinations and investigations by physicians. Most of these symptoms are temporary and go away on their own.

By contrast, research has shown that at as many as 3 in 100 will suffer from chronic, persistent, disabling physical problems for which no specific cause can be identified. Most of these cases turn out to be the result of Somatoform Disorders.

Up to one-third of patients with a previously diagnosed medical or neurological problem (such as multiple sclerosis or epilepsy) may repeatedly show symptoms that are not part of that medical problem.

What causes them?

Somatization may occur in milder forms that include common stress reactions such as headaches, neck and shoulder muscle tension, mild stomach or bowel problems, and fatigue. Mild symptoms typically go away as the stress eases. Physicians understand the symptoms as due to dysregulated and excessive autonomic (automatic and involuntary) nervous system activity.

When symptoms are more long-term and disabling, the patient's psychological problems may be much more complex. These problems are often linked to more serious underlying psychiatric conditions. Most patients are not aware of their distress or of the illness that lies behind their physical problems. This is because the process is unconscious. These patients do not choose to be ill, and they are not "faking it." They don't recognize the connection between their emotional and physical experiences and misattribute physical symptoms commonly and understandably to disease and not emotional distress.

Since patients with undiagnosed Somatoform Disorders do not know what is causing their symptoms, they look to their family doctors, specialists, or alternative practitioners for explanations. This may lead to unnecessary procedures, investigations, and treatments. These treatments put patients at higher risk for side effects or other complications, and they delay the correct treatment of the real problem.

Some patients are very sensitive to changes in their bodies. These patients are more likely to misinterpret sensations caused by strong emotions and stressful events. These patients often have difficulty recognizing and expressing their feelings.
Stressful life situations may contribute to the onset of Somatoform Disorders. For example, people who have been hurt emotionally, physically, or sexually are at higher risk.

Somatoform Disorders may also follow accidents, surgery, side effects of medications, or illnesses.

Do depression and anxiety cause somatization?

Stress and/or a chemical imbalance in the brain can cause impaired brain function, which can lead to depression and anxiety. If depression and anxiety are not treated, somatization may develop.

How is the diagnosis confirmed?

To ensure there are no other serious health problems, the psychiatrist, together with the family doctor and other specialists, will complete an in-depth assessment. There is no specific test for somatization. The first step toward a diagnosis involves looking for clues that the process is in fact emotionally based and not due to disease, and at the same time ruling out any other conditions or diseases.
This is done through:

- Talking and analyzing the problems and symptoms
- A physical examination
- A review of tests

Somatization can be made worse by difficulties with thinking and processing emotional information. For this reason, patients may be referred to a psychologist for testing. With our current medical knowledge, proper psychiatric evaluation, and advanced testing techniques (e.g. CT and MRI scans), it is very rare for a serious physical illness to be overlooked.

In these disorders, as with any other health issue, new symptoms often appear. The family doctor and psychiatrist will address these symptoms promptly to figure out whether they are due to somatization or due to a new health problem.

What will the doctor recommend?

Experience suggests that a supportive doctor who understands the complexity of the problem should see patients regularly. When chronic, disabling, unexplained physical symptoms develop, a referral to a psychiatrist should be made.
The first goal is an in-depth understanding of the nature and origin of the symptoms. This may be the most important intervention, and it may be enough to cause the symptoms to go away.

Medications are often of great benefit. Studies show that antidepressants and other medications that improve the proper function of the brain and the nervous system can reverse symptoms—sometimes dramatically.

Opiates (narcotic pain killers such as morphine) and other habit-forming medications will not cure these disorders. These medications mask the psychiatric symptoms and produce disabling side effects such as constipation, sleepiness, and memory problems, in addition to making it more challenging for individuals to identify and manage the emotional distress causing the somatization.

What else can be done?

Even though patients do not play an active role in the development of the illness, there is much they can do to aid in their recovery. Activities such as regular exercise and social events, occupational therapy, physiotherapy, massage therapy, acupuncture, and biofeedback may be helpful. These options should be discussed with the doctor.

Most people will improve with talk therapies (i.e., psychotherapy). Psychotherapy helps patients:

- Understand the nature of their condition
- Correctly identify bodily signals caused by strong emotions
- Build their emotional ability to recover from difficult events
- Build their problem-solving skills to help them deal more effectively with stress and other emotions

Do people with these disorders get better?

Somatization that has been present for a few weeks or months tends to go away on its own or with simple treatments. Symptoms of somatization that have lasted for many months or years are much more difficult to treat.

No matter how long the symptoms last, most patients will benefit from treatment.

With treatment, some can expect their symptoms to disappear. Others may still have symptoms but will be able to function better.

At times, these disorders may come back months or years later. Fortunately, symptoms rarely return to their previous level, because a greater understanding of the condition then leads to timely appropriate treatment.

LETTER TO DSM-5 WORKING GROUP

UBC Neuropsychiatry Unit

28 June 2011

To: DSM-5 Somatic Symptom Disorders Work Group
Dimsdale, Joel E., M.D.
Barsky III, Arthur J., M.D.
Creed, Francis, M.D.
Frasure-Smith, Nancy, Ph.D.
Irwin, Michael R., M.D.
Keefe, Francis J., Ph.D.
Lee, Sing, M.D.
Levenson, James L., M.D.
Sharpe, Michael, M.D.
Wulsin, Lawson R., M.D.

Dear Members of the DSM-5 Somatic Symptom Disorders Work Group:

Re: Somatoform Disorders; Somatic Symptom Disorders; Intended DSM-5 Changes

We are a group of clinicians who treat individuals suffering from neuropsychiatric conditions. Most of us have a background in general psychiatry with subspecialization in neuropsychiatry. We work together as a team practising both inpatient and outpatient neuropsychiatry at UBC Hospital, University of British Columbia, Vancouver, Canada. A significant part of our work, up to 40% of our clinical time, is spent treating individuals suffering from severe somatoform disorders. We each have between 5 and 22 years of experience working with this population.

We note the invitation for readers of the DSM-5 website to review and comment on the proposed DSM-5 organizational structure and criteria changes, and we welcome the opportunity to do so regarding Somatoform Disorders.

We would at the outset like to thank you all for the amount of work that you are doing in your efforts to improve the Somatoform Disorders diagnostic category.

We know as well as you how prevalent these disorders are, and we are acutely aware of the very significant burden of suffering that is borne by patients suffering from these disorders. We share your determination to help this group of individuals in the future, and it is in this spirit that we share our thoughts with you.

DSM-IV's handling of Somatoform Disorders without doubt led to extreme under-diagnosis, caused clinicians and patients to shun these diagnoses, and deterred much needed research. We are in agreement with you that the classification of this category of disorders requires revision, and we have studied the changes you are suggesting in your latest drafts and discussion documents. ['*Somatic Symptom Disorders*' (DRAFT April 18, 2011) and '*Justification of Criteria – Somatic Symptoms*' (DRAFT 4/18/11)]

We applaud your suggestions regarding the collapsing of Somatization Disorder, Hypochondriasis, Undifferentiated Somatoform Disorder and Pain Disorder into a single continuum. This makes excellent sense. In fact, it could be argued that there is a place for going further, and to collapse Conversion Disorder, too, into that continuum (but continuing to differentiate it somehow by symptom type).

We do, however, have concerns about the very major changes you are suggesting regarding the criteria for the resulting continuum/syndrome (CSSD/SSSD), and the proposed name for the entire category of disorders.

Here are our concerns about the changes you are contemplating:

1. We disagree with the suggested abandonment of the idea of 'medically unexplained symptoms'.

You argue that using 'medically unexplained symptoms' as a defining feature of these disorders "*enforces a dualism between psychiatric and medical conditions*", "*bases a diagnosis on a negative*", and "*runs the risk of misdiagnosis*".

We would argue that using 'medically unexplained symptoms' as a criteria to classify somatoform disorders is of central importance. We believe that there is overwhelming evidence that a valid syndrome (or group of syndromes) exists where symptoms and signs do not follow known disease patterns, and where investigations reveal no evidence of 'general medical' disease. These conditions are likely but not unequivocally the result of emotional distress being expressed as physical symptoms, through the process widely referred to as 'somatization'. (A causative theory for 'medically unexplained symptoms' need not be part of the criteria used for a somatoform syndrome).
Your proposed attempt to move away from the concept of 'medically unexplained symptoms' will, we believe, discard a very valid distinction, and result in 'somatoform disorders' being lost in a broader and less clearly valid syndrome. This will profoundly alter how clinicians, patients and researchers conceptualize these disorders and, we respectfully submit our belief that this change will be a grave classification error. 'Somatoform Disorders' will be diluted and lost in the broader SSD classification, and we fear that clinical and research advances will be slowed or arrested.

Regarding your concern that 'medically unexplained symptoms' as a term "*enforces a dualism between psychiatric and medical conditions*": As we are all aware, our field has been wrestling with dualism for decades. The concept of somatoform disorders may evoke dualistic thinking in some clinicians and patients by virtue of the fact that these disorders involve both complex mind/brain processes and seemingly more straightforward physical symptoms. This dualistic thinking is, needless to say, incorrect.
All neuropsychiatric conditions are mediated by brain function. All aspects of somatoform disorders are a product of complex brain function

and dysfunction, the specific nature of which we do not yet understand. To further our understanding of the neurobiology of these conditions, it is absolutely vital that we address the challenge presented by the common tendency to dualistic thinking. The answer is not to abandon the concept of somatoform disorders because of this common tendency. The correct path forward is to wrestle with the challenge, to engage the field in discussion, and to educate clinicians and patients about the 'bridging' nature of these conditions; they involve brain/mind/body. A thorough understanding of the concept of somatoform processes can actually be an integrative force in this regard. [See our further relevant discussion below regarding nomenclature.]
Abandoning 'medically unexplained symptoms' as a term for fear of common misconceptions about the concept makes little sense. We should rather retain the term and put effort into educating those ignorant of these nuances.

Regarding your concerns that use of the concept of 'medically unexplained symptoms' is flawed because it *"bases a diagnosis on a negative"*: Clinicians go through a process of elimination whenever they consider the differential diagnosis for any set of symptoms and signs. Exclusion of known diseases is part of every diagnostic process. If, at the end of such a process, the clinical picture suggests 'medically unexplained symptoms', then they should be called that. That judgment is not qualitatively different from what we are doing with all other disease entities.

It is also implied (and specifically stated in some of the literature that you reference) that making the diagnosis of a 'Somatoform Disorder' is somehow a 'negative' step in a broader sense, in that clinicians and patients see it as the 'taking away' of something rather than a 'positive' diagnosis.

We would argue that making a 'somatoform disorder' diagnosis is as proactive a diagnostic step as the making of any other diagnosis, and we believe that we in the field should work to actively frame it as such. The patient should be informed that their syndrome is the result of complex brain and mind processes, not demonstrable brain or peripheral tissue pathology. This has positive implications for treatment, and we help the patient understand that.

Many diagnoses in general medicine embrace the fact that there are unknown components to the pathogenesis. After ruling out hypertension secondary to renal, endocrine, or other general medical conditions, the hypertension is labeled 'idiopathic'. Patients don't commonly complain that they have lost something or had something 'taken away' in that process.

Regarding your concerns that use of the concept of 'medically unexplained symptoms' is flawed because it *"runs the risk of misdiagnosis"*:
Clinicians need, after very thorough assessment, to make a judgment call about whether the symptoms and signs at hand follow the patterns of known diseases. If they do not, then they should conclude that the condition is 'somatoform'. Thorough clinical assessment, and the diagnostic tools available to us circa 2011, allow clinicians to make such judgments at an acceptable level of accuracy. This level of accuracy likely compares with those levels of reliability reached with other psychiatric conditions, and, indeed, with many general medical condition diagnoses. In fact, we would suggest that it is the clinician's *duty* to make such judgments and to offer to treat the patient accordingly. It is only with such a judgment call that appropriate management can be instituted. This is the approach that we would request for ourselves, or our loved ones, if we were suffering from these conditions.
Making this judgment may be challenging, and, inter-rater reliability may be imperfect, but that is not reason to abandon the concept or this approach. As a group, clinicians and researchers in this area need to put effort into testing reliability, improving our assessment approaches, and perhaps even attempt to standardize ways of making these judgments, rather than abandoning this aspect of the diagnostic process.
Pointing to suboptimal inter-rater reliability is not a reason to discard the core concept in the understanding of these conditions.

Thus, our overall position regarding the issue of 'medically unexplained symptoms' is that we do not believe that it is correct or beneficial for clinicians to abdicate their responsibility to their patients and to stop making this diagnostic distinction.
Identifying 'medically unexplained symptoms' (or whatever term we want to use for the concept) remains central to the diagnosis of these disorders, and we should retain that concept in future classification systems.

2. If you do abandon 'medically unexplained symptoms', we have concerns regarding the threshold for diagnosis of CSSD/SSSD:

As it is, about 16%-20% of patients in primary care waiting rooms around the world appear to meet criteria for a somatoform disorder. By dropping the threshold of entry into this group we will now have a very large number of people meeting criteria for Somatic Symptom Disorders (SSDs), either CSSD or SSSD, who did not previously meet criteria for Somatoform Disorder. SSDs will now include all individuals who have a physical symptom due to tissue pathology who show 'excessive' concern about the symptom.

Our concern is that there will now be substantially more individuals getting these diagnoses. We would not be surprised if numbers go as high as 40% or 50% of individuals in a primary care waiting room, who have, after all, already selected themselves by being 'concerned' about one or another symptom.

This is alarming, as it will have two effects:

(a) It will dilute out individuals with 'true' Somatoform conditions. They will be lost in the noise of patients excessively concerned with symptoms of physical illness (a valid but *different* concern);

and, perhaps more important,

(b) The condition will become so common as to be rendered meaningless and thus useless to patients and clinicians.

3. We have concerns regarding the chosen nomenclature:

We are very concerned that the suggested name, 'Somatic Symptom Disorders' is flawed. It is not descriptively accurate, in the most straightforward sense, as it implies that the category includes all disorders with 'somatic symptoms'. The vast majority of general medical conditions result in 'somatic symptoms', and thus they are, from a purely descriptive perspective, 'somatic symptom disorders'. Calling previously named 'somatoform' conditions 'Somatic Symptom Disorders' will lead to ambiguity and confusion. We strongly believe this term is *worse* than maintaining the name 'Somatoform Disorders'.

We particularly like 'Somatoform' as a name: it implies that the disorders are 'in the form of the body' (while at the same time implying that their cause is more complex). 'Somatoform' disorders are 'of the body' AND 'of the mind'. The word embraces integration. It implies a holistic approach.

Even if the term, up to this point, may not have been understood in this way by all clinicians and patients, it is our job as psychiatrists to educate our colleagues and our patients in this regard.
Similar battles are being successfully fought regarding educating clinicians and patients about other terms deemed unpalatable to some, for example: 'psychosis'. We would be amiss to avoid the most appropriate term for a condition, in the interest of short-term palatability gains, but at substantial cost to validity and accuracy.

We would thus suggest retaining the name 'Somatoform Disorders' for the DSM 5 classification system; that would be our preference. Alternatively we'd recommend use of another term that embraces the fact that these conditions are the result of physical symptom manifestations of complex brain/mind mechanisms.
Other possible names that may embrace the concept adequately could be 'Psychogenic Somatic Symptom Disorders', or 'Psychosomatic Disorders'.

4. We would caution against using administrative or political considerations in deciding how to classify these disorders.

Conditions should *not* be grouped together:
- because patients with these conditions tend to be seen in similar clinics
- because, thus far, they tend to get similar treatments
- in order to encourage multidisciplinary collaboration

This is all 'cart-before-horse' logic, and threatens to decrease syndrome validity.
All efforts should be put into classifying syndromes according to probable underlying pathogenetic/pathophysiological factors.
Political and administrative considerations are important but, for the purpose of disorder classification, they must be secondary to the attempts to find the most neurobiologically valid syndromes.

We have numerous lesser concerns, and will not list them here; many are moot if the major concerns raised above were addressed.

We hope that our thoughts and concerns above will be helpful in your ongoing deliberations. We trust, too, that our thoughts are taken in the spirit of constructive criticism in which they are intended.
We would be happy to engage in dialogue with you about any of these

suggestions if that may be helpful.

We wish you well in the daunting task of improving this section of the DSM.

Sincerely,

Anton Scamvougeras, MBChB, FRCPC (Neuropsychiatrist)
Leon Berzen, MBBCh, FFPsych(SA), FRCPC (Neuropsychiatrist)
Joseph Tham BMc, MD, FRCPC (Neuropsychiatrist)
Andrew Howard MD, FRCPC (Neuropsychiatrist)
Magda Ilcewicz MD, FRCPC (Neuropsychiatrist)
Marius Dimov MD, FRCPC (Neuropsychiatrist)
Robert Stowe MD, FRCPS, UCNS (Behavioural Neurologist)
Trevor Hurwitz MBChB, MRCP(UK), FRCP (Neurologist & Psychiatrist)

All above are members of:
UBC Neuropsychiatry Unit
University of British Columbia
Vancouver, BC
Canada

INDEX